JOHN EBNEZAR CBS | Handbooks in
Orthopedics and Fractures

SERIES

Orthopedic Trauma

# Sports Injuries

VOLUME II

- Lower Limb Injuries in Sports
- Spinal Injuries in Sports

## John Ebnezar

- Holder of the **Guinness Book of World Records** for the most number of books written by an individual in a single year.
- Listed in the **India Book of Records** for the most number of books written by an individual.
- Recipient of the highest civilian awards of Karnataka, the **Rajyotsava Award 2010** and the **Kempegowda Award 2011**.
- Recipient of the **Best Citizen of India Award** by the International Publishing house.
- Former Vice-President, the Indian Orthopaedic Association
- President, Neuro-Spinal Surgeons Association of India (Karnataka)
- CEO, Parimala Health Care Services, A ISO 9001:2008 Hospital, Bilekahalli, Bannerghatta Road, Bangalore
- Ebnezar Orthopedic Center, Bilekahalli, Bannerghatta Road, Bangalore
- Dr John's Orthopedic Clinic, near Reliance Mart, Arakere, BG Road, Bangalore
- Chairman, the Physically Handicapped and Paraplegic Charitable Trust of Karnataka®
- Founder President, Geriatric Orthopedic Society
- Founder President, Orthopedic Authors Association and All India Medical Authors Association
- Chairman, Karnataka Orthopedic Academy®
- President, Bangalore Holistic Academy
- Chairman, Rakesh Cultural Academy
- President, Vaidya Kala Ranga, Bangalore
- Secretary, SK Educational Society®
- Former Senior Specialist, Victoria Hospital, Bangalore Medical College, Bangalore
- Former Assistant Professor in Orthopedics, Devaraj Urs Medical College, Kolar, Karnataka
- Postgraduate teacher, Bangalore Baptist Hospital, Airport Road, Bangalore

John Ebnezar CBS | Handbooks in Orthopedics and Fractures

SERIES

Orthopedic Trauma

# Sports Injuries

**Volume II**

- Lower Limb Injuries in Sports
- Spinal Injuries in Sports

**John Ebnezar**

MBBS, D'Ortho, DNB (Ortho), MNAMS (Ortho), PhD (Yoga)
Sports Medicine (Australia), INOR Fellow (UK), DAc, DMT

Consulting Orthopedic and Spine Surgeon,
Holistic Orthopedic Expert, and Sports Specialist
Bangalore

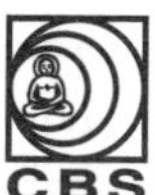

CBS Publishers & Distributors Pvt Ltd
New Delhi • Bengaluru • Pune • Kochi • Chennai

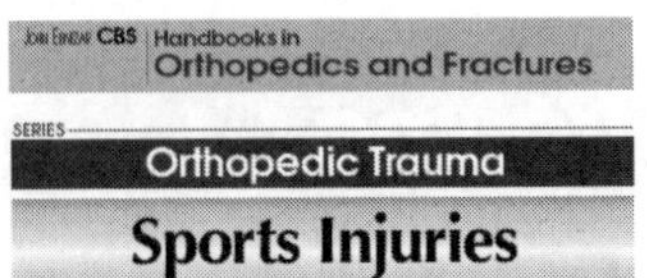


ISBN: 978-81-239-2102-0



**First Edition:** 2012



Published by Satish Kumar Jain and produced by Vinod K. Jain for
**CBS Publishers & Distributors** Pvt Ltd
4819/XI Prahlad Street, 24 Ansari Road, Daryaganj
New Delhi 110 002, India.
Ph: 23289259, 23266861, 23266867
Fax: 011-23243014
Website: www.cbspd.com
e-mail: delhi@cbspd.com
cbspubs@airtelmail.in.

*Branches*

- Bengaluru: Seema House 2975, 17th Cross, K.R. Road, Banasankari 2nd Stage, Bengaluru 560 070, Karnataka
  Ph: +91-80-26771678/79 Fax: +91-80-26771680 e-mail: bangalore@cbspd.com
- Pune: Bhuruk Prestige, Sr. No. 52/12/2+1+3/2 Narhe, Haveli (Near Katraj-Dehu Road Bypass), Pune 411 051, Maharashtra
  Ph: 020-64704058, 64704059, 32392277 Fax: +91-020-24300160 e-mail: pune@cbspd.com
- Kochi: 36/14 Kalluvilakam, Lissie Hospital Road, Kochi 682 018, Kerala
  Ph: +91-484-4059061-65 Fax: +91-484-4059065 e-mail: cochin@cbspd.com
- Chennai: 20, West Park Road, Shenoy Nagar, Chennai 600 030, Tamil Nadu
  Ph: +91-44-26260666, 26208620 Fax: +91-44-45530020 email: chennai@cbspd.com

*Printed at* Magic International, Greater Noida (UP)

*to*

---

*my mother*
*(late) Sampath Kumari*
*who taught me that life is more than self and*
*there is more joy in giving and sharing than taking*

*my wife*
*Dr Parimala*

*my lovely children*
*Rakesh and Priyanka*
*who are an epitome of love, sacrifice, encouragement*
*and inspiration*

*all my teachers*
*who made me what I am today*

*all my students*
*past and present*

*and*

*all my patients*

**Dr John Ebnezar**

is a legendary name as a prolific orthopedic writer. No other orthopedic surgeon in the world has come anywhere close to him in the number of books he has written in his field. He is the first orthopedic surgeon in the world to be listed in the **Guinness Book of World Records** for the most number of books written by an individual in a single year. For the same feat his name has been listed in the **India Book of Records.** This book, like all his previous books, carries his flavor of simple and lucid writing, excellent language, beautiful illustrations and excellent presentation of the topics. This book is a part of the 100+ book series he has brought out in a single calendar year of 2012 on a wide array of orthopedic problems of public health importance. No other individual in the world has brought out these many books in one year and this is a world record attempt. With these books he aims to educate the reader and the public about these common orthopedic problems.

All his books have been accepted very well and he has a great fan following all over the world. He has been bestowed with as many as 32 international, national and state awards including Karnataka state's highest civilian award the **Rajyotsava Award 2010** and the **Kempegowda Award 2011,** apart from the **Best Citizen of India Award** given by the International Publishing House. He is the pioneer in holistic orthopedics and is credited for discovering a new method of treatment for the common orthopedic problems and has done PhD in arthritis from the world famous S-VYASA University, Bangalore. He is currently president of the Neuro-Spinal Surgeons Association of India (Karnataka), the former Vice-President of the Indian Orthopedic Association, and is the founder president of various orthopedic bodies.

# Preface

This book is a part of the 100+ book series

**JOHN EBNEZAR CBS Handbooks in Orthopedics and Fractures**

which deals with the orthopedic problems of public health importance. The purpose of these books is to educate and create awareness among the readers about various problems associated with orthopedics. Through this way the readers get to know all about various orthopedic problems directly from a specialist. This will help a reader immensely in getting the right knowledge as most of them depend on the internet and magazines which distort and misrepresent various pieces of information concerning health topics, leaving the readers confused and worse still improperly educated. This may harm more than helping them find solutions to their problems. The purpose of these books, therefore, is to educate the readers right in their quest for knowledge on the common health and associated problems.

The 100+ book series has been brought out in a single calendar year.

Sports as a career is being considered by a vast majority of people in recent times It is no more a taboo as a profession thanks to the encouragement, support earning opportunities and fame associated with most of the sports like cricket, tennis, badminton, athletics, etc. As more and more people are taking up sports, sports related problems are on the rise. Among the various sports related problems, orthopedic injuries associated with sports are seeing an increasing trend. Orthopedic related sports injuries can range from a minor strain to sprain or to a major fracture and dislocation of any of the bone or joints. Diagnosis and managing them is quite a challenge as unlike in a general population, a sportsperson needs to get back to the sporting action fast. For this to happen, diagnosis and treatment have to be perfect and most importantly the rehabilitation program has to be very good. The career of a sportsman is short and any error or mismanagement of sports related orthopedic injury can prematurely cut short their professional life. Hence it is of paramount important to tackle sports related injuries effectively. This book enables the reader to have a glimpse about all the issues related to sports injuries. As with all the books in these series, this book also aims to educate the reader and create awareness about sports related orthopedic injuries.

This is the first ever book which exclusively deals with the orthopedic sports injuries and I have made an attempt to bring all the important basic aspects about it in one book, so that the reader gets to know about them.

***Highlights of this book***

- Simple and lucid language
- Good illustrations
- Good clinical photographs wherever necessary
- Relevant X-rays
- Short summaries
- Anecdotes

This book has ubiquitous utility and usage and can be useful to the orthopedic surgeons, postgraduate students in orthopedics, undergraduate medical students, doctors from all disciplines of medicine, physiotherapists, therapists practising alternative systems of medicine, rehabilitation specialists, and most importantly the common people. It is particularly useful to those unsung heroes who work in remote areas with minimum infrastructure. They can use this book as a ready-reckoner. Seldom will you find a book that covers such a wide spectrum of readers.

Knowing all about the sports injuries creates awareness and helps one to understand them well and thereby prevent complications from happening.

Constructive criticism and useful suggestions are invited to make the book more effective in its forthcoming editions.

**John Ebnezar**

# Acknowledgments

This volume is a part of the 100+ book series brought out in a single calendar year. This was a huge and mammoth task attempted first time ever by an author and a publisher in the world. Such an herculean effort could not have been possible without the active involvement of those concerned in CBS Publishers & Distributors. I thank Mr Satish K Jain, Managing Director of CBS P&D, for agreeing to be a part of this world-record feat in bringing out this book in the Series. My special thanks to Mr YN Arjuna who showed special interest in this work and channelized his entire energy into this improbable feat. My special thanks to Mrs Ritu Chawla and her entire dedicated team who have toiled day and night to make this dream a reality. I thank members of the entire editorial–production team of CBS P&D who have worked hard behind the scenes to bring out this book.

My special thanks to Dr Yogitha for actively helping me in the compilation of all the books. I also thank all the staff members of my hospital who have helped me at various levels during the making of this book.

**John Ebnezar**

# Contents

John Ebnezar CBS | Handbooks in
# Orthopedics and Fractures

**TITLES IN THE SERIES**

## I Orthopedic Trauma

*General Fractures*

1 General Principles of Fractures and Dislocations
2 Fracture Treatment Methods
3 Fractures and their Complications
4 Atypical Fractures

*Injuries of Upper Limb*

5 Injuries of Shoulder
6 Injuries of Arm
7 Injuries of Elbow
8 Injuries of Forearm
9 Injuries of Wrist and Hand
10 Injuries of Distal Forearm and Wrist
11 Injuries of Hand
12 Injuries of Upper Limb

*Injuries of Lower Limb*

13 Injuries of Hip
14 Injuries of Femur
15 Injuries of Knee
16 Injuries of Knee and Leg
17 Injuries of Ankle and Leg
18 Injuries of Foot and Ankle
19 Injuries of Lower Limb

*Injuries of Axial Skeleton*

20 Injuries of Pelvis and Hip
21 Injuries of Spine
22 Injuries of Pelvis and Spine

23 Sports Injuries Volume I
24 Sports Injuries Volume II
25 Soft Tissue Problems in Orthopedics
26 Geriatric Trauma
27 Pediatric Trauma

## II Orthopedic Disease

28 Congenital Orthopedic Problems
29 Developmental Orthopedic Problems

## III Specific Orthopedic Problems



## IV Regional Orthopedic Problems



## V Orthopedic Injuries and Surgeries

*Upper Limb*



*Lower Limb*

## VI Practical Examination



## VII Orthopedic Problems of Different Ages



## VIII Common Orthopedic Problems

## IX Yoga Therapy in Common Orthopedic Problems

1

# Lower Limb Injuries in Sports

## Introduction

Lower limb injuries are very common in sports. It may be minor strains to major fractures. Knee injuries, ankle injuries are more commonly seen. Sports related lower limb injuries keep the sportsperson and athletes out of action for weeks and in some extreme situations may be the end of their carrier in sports. This managing the lower limb sports injuries are challenging. The following are the common lower limb injuries in sports.

### *Hip and Pelvis*

- Piriformis syndrome
- Iliotibial tract syndrome
- Glutei bursitis
- Trochanteric bursitis.

### *Knee and Leg*

- Collateral ligament injury
- Cruciate ligament injury
- Meniscal injury
- Quadriceps strain
- Hamstrings strain
- Calf muscle strain
- Patellar tendonitis
- Plica syndrome

*Ankle and Foot*

- Ankle sprain
- Plantar fasciitis
- Tendo-Achilles injuries
- Tarsal tunnel syndrome

Now let us know some of the important sports injuries of the lower limbs.

## KNEE LIGAMENT INJURIES (COMMON)

### GENERAL PRINCIPLES

#### Etiology

- *Athletes:* Knee ligament injuries are very common in athletes who are involved both in contact and non-contact sports. The injury could be either direct due to the collision with another athlete or indirect due to rotation and twisting injuries.
- *Road traffic accident (RTA):* Here the mechanism is usually direct and could be due to a dashboard injury.
- *Fall* from a height with twisting force.

#### Mechanism of Injury (Palmar)

The following are the common mechanism of knee ligament injuries (Fig. 1.1):

- Direct valgus (outward) force.
- Rotational or twisting forces.
  - *Abduction, flexion and internal rotation of femur on tibia (Ab FIR):* This causes damage to medial structures, like tibial collateral, medial capsule and if more force is applied ACL and medial meniscus may also tear.
    *"O'Donoghue's unhappy triad"* (Fig. 1.2): Indicate injuries to medial structures + ACL tear + medial meniscus injury.
  - *Adduction, flexion and external rotation of femur on tibia (Ad FER):* Causes damage to fibular collateral, lateral

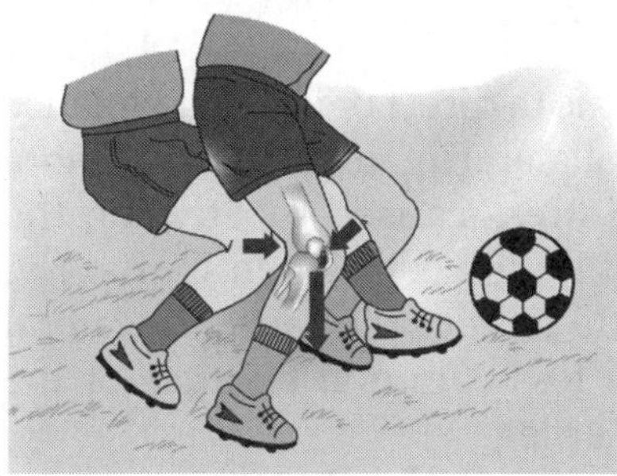

**Fig. 1.1:** Common mechanism of knee ligament injuries in contact sports

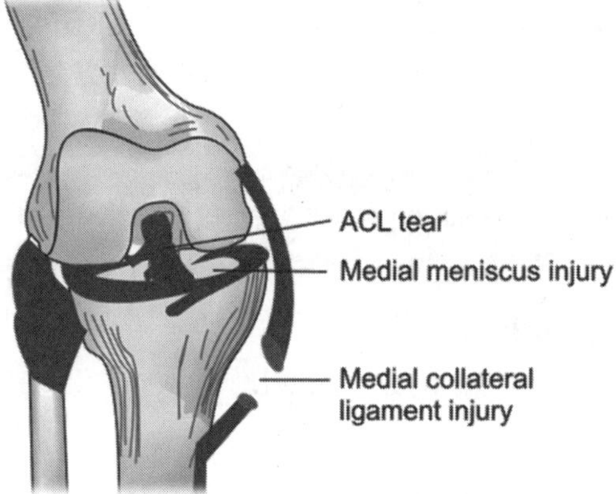


**Fig. 1.2:** Here three structures of the knee are injured and is called unhappy triad of O'Donoghue

capsule, arcuate complex, popliteus, iliotibial band, biceps, common peroneal nerve, anterior, posterior or both cruciates.

- *Hyperextension force* may cause either anterior or posterior cruciate ligament injury.
- *Anteroposterior displacement* either anterior (dashboard injury) or posterior cruciates may be injured due to a direct force in RTA.

## What are the Goals of Treatment?

The goals of treatment in knee ligament injuries are restoration of anatomy and stability to normal or near to normal as possible.

## COLLATERAL LIGAMENT INJURY

Collateral ligament injury is due to direct or indirect violence as described earlier. Medial collateral ligament injury is more common due to the valgus stress caused by striking the lateral aspect of the knee joint during collision in sports. The varus force on the medial side required to cause the lateral collateral ligament injury is less common because of the protection offered by the other leg.

However, a severe varus force may cause avulsion of the lateral collateral ligament from the head of the fibula (Fig. 1.3A).

> **Do you know?**
>
> About Pellegrini-Stieda disease: It is a calcification seen at the adductor tubercle visualized on AP X-ray of the knee in MCL injury of greater than 6 weeks.

### Mechanism of Injury

This has already been described.

### Types

Depending upon on the degree of tear collateral ligament injuries are graded into three types (Flow chart 1.1 and Fig. 1.3B)

**Flow chart 1.1:** Classification (American Medical Association)

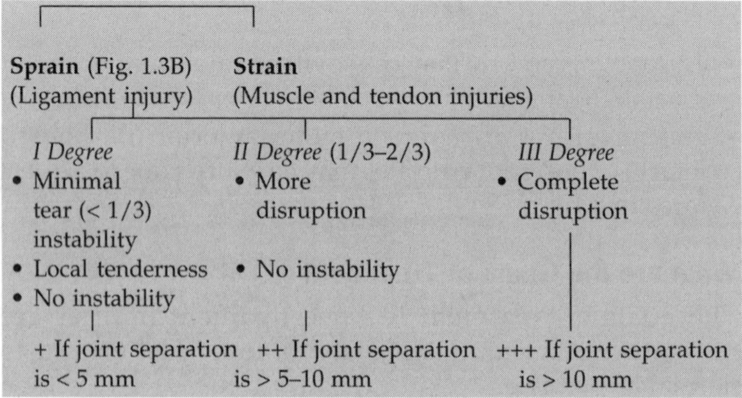

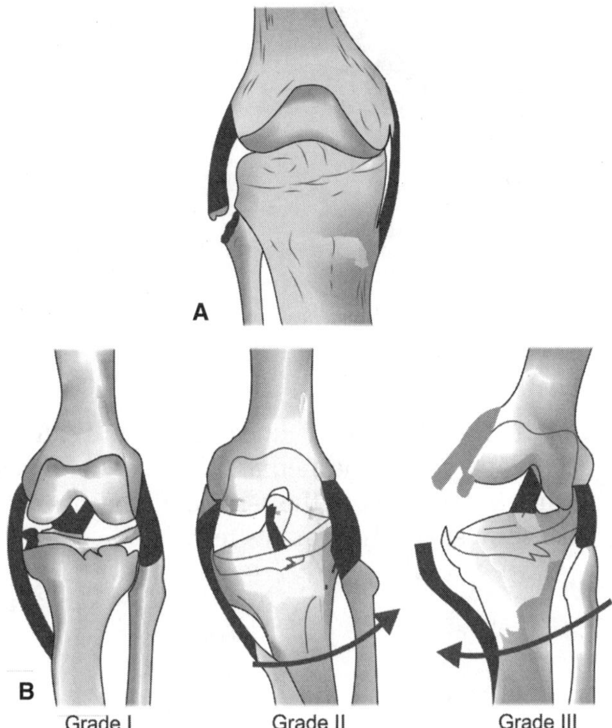


**Figs 1.3A and B:** (A) Avulsion of lateral collateral ligament from the head of the fibula, and (B) Sprain of medial collateral ligament of the knee

## Clinical Features

The patient gives history of valgus and external rotation force in mild sprains. In severe sprains, the patient gives history of valgus stress force due to the direct blow on the lower thigh or upper leg seen commonly in contact sports like football, rugby, etc. It may be associated with ACL tear or meniscal injury and then the patient may present with pain, swelling, hemarthrosis, etc.

On examination, the point of local tenderness could be at adductor tubercle, joint line or at the insertion of tibial collateral ligament (Fig. 1.4). About 10–20 percent of patients have damage to the extensor mechanism of the knee.

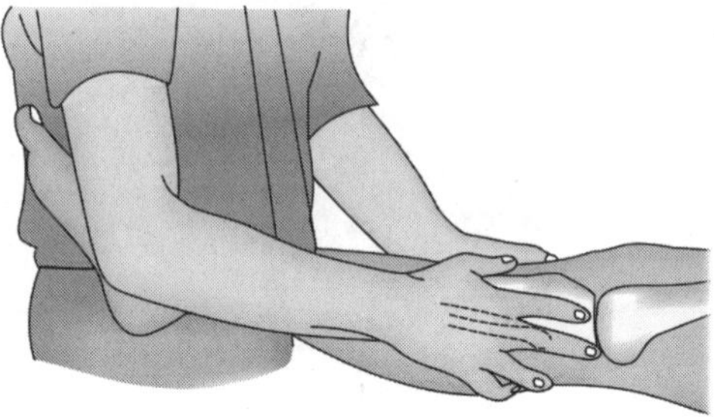

**Fig. 1.4:** Method of eliciting joint line tenderness

## Clinical Tests

These are abduction stress in 30° knee flexion and extension. The amount of opening on the medial side should be assessed (Figs 1.5A and B). To rule out the associated injuries, do the anterior drawer test and Lachman's test.

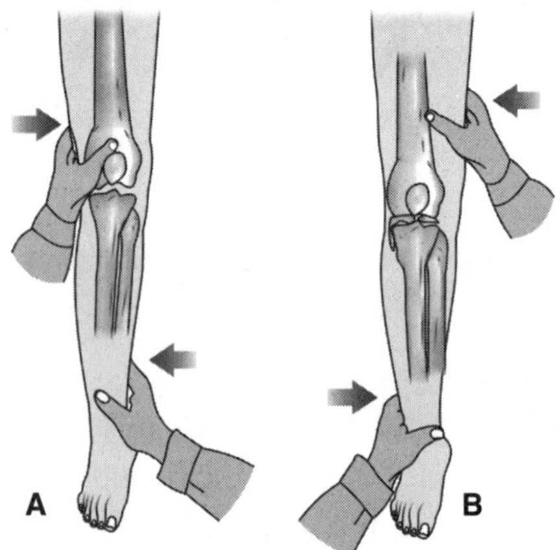


**Figs 1.5A and B:** Stress tests: (A) Abduction or valgus stress test, and (B) Adduction or varus stress test

## Investigations

- Stress radiographs at 15–20° of valgus.
- MRI helps to localize the MCL tears, ACL, meniscal injuries, etc.

- Arthrograms and arthroscopy to evaluate and rule out meniscal and cruciate pathology.

## Treatment

Fresh injury nonoperative treatment is the mainstay of treatment.

I° Sprain →symptomatic treatment, nonsteroidal anti-inflammatory drugs (NSAIDs), etc.

II° Sprain →long leg cast for 4-6 weeks with knee in 30–40° of flexion.

III° Sprain →surgical repair in isolated tears. Repair and reconstruction in old tears or in associated injuries (Fig. 1.6). Brace is required for 4–7 months.

### *Old Cases*

Here surgery is the main stay of treatment and consists of mainly reconstruction.

*Tibial collateral ligament (TCL) injury:* If TCL is intact but lax, then distal transfer is done. If ligament is destroyed, reconstruction using hamstrings or semitendinosus is done.

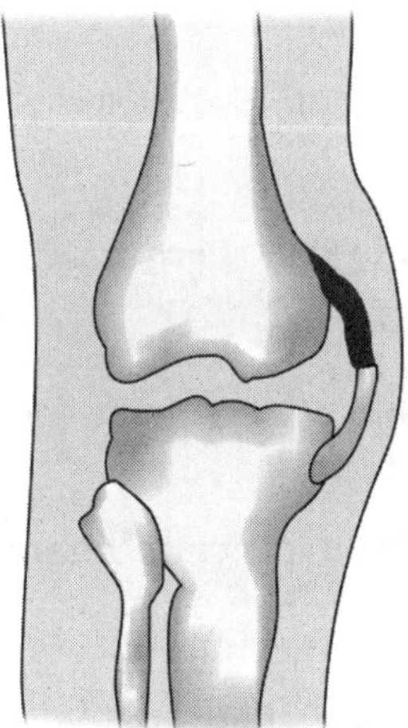

**Fig. 1.6:** Direct ligament repair in fresh tears

*Fibular collateral ligament injury:* If adequate and thick, distal transfer is recommended. If destroyed, reconstruction using fascia lata, biceps tendon, etc. is done.

## CRUCIATE LIGAMENT INJURIES

### ANTERIOR CRUCIATE LIGAMENT (ACL) TEAR

Of all the knee ligament injuries, ACL tear is the most common (Fig. 1.7).

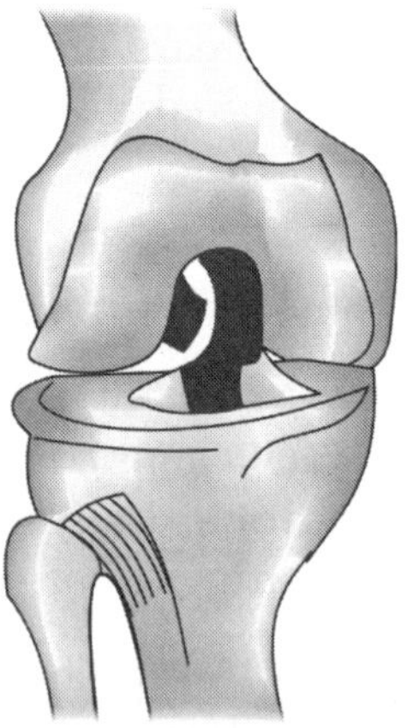

**Fig. 1.7:** ACL tear

**Know the role of ACL in your knees**

- AP stability
- Proprioception
- Mechanical function

**Mechanism** of anterior cruciate ligament (ACL) tear has already been discussed. The most common mode of injury is external rotation with abduction of the flexed knee or hyperextension of knee in internal rotation. This is a disabling injury and the knee may immediately collapse and is painful.

### Clinical Features

Popping sensation felt or heard at the time of injury signifies ligamentous injury (ACL tear). The patient also tells that the knee "gave away" or buckled at the time of injury. Swelling of the knee could be either due to hemarthroses or traumatic synovitis and the distended knee is held in partial flexion by the hamstrings (*see* box for differential diagnosis).

*Note:* Sixty-seven percent of ACL tear is sports related.

**Quick facts: ACL tear**

Differential diagnosis: Hemarthrosis

- Ligamentous tears (ACL, PCL, etc.)
- Osteochondral fracture
- Peripheral menisci tear
- Capsular tear
- Patellar dislocation
- Intra-articular fractures

*Note:* Commonest cause is ACL tear.

**Did you know?**

Galen first described ACL tear in AD 170.

### Clinical Examination

Always examine the normal knee first and form a basis for "comparison". Clinical findings depend on associated ligamentous injury or meniscal injury or bone damage. Depending on the combination, there will be specific instabilities (Table 1.1) that will allow anterior displacement of tibia on the uninvolved side. Anterior subluxation of more than 5° suggests lax or disrupted ACL. Isolated injury is rare. Anterior drawer test and Lachman's test are specific to ACL tear and various other clinical tests to detect ACL tear are depicted in Table 1.1 and Fig 1.8A to F.

**Table 1.1:** Clinical tests to diagnose various knee ligament injuries

| *Tests* | *How to perform* | *Inference* |
|---|---|---|
| **Adduction or varus: Abduction or valgus stress test** (Fig. 1.8A) 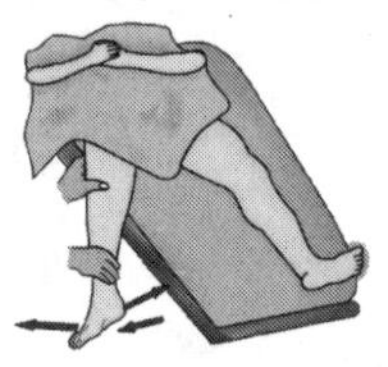 **Fig. 1.8A** | Patient is supine, knee is flexed to 30° **For abduction test:** One hand is on the lateral aspect of the knee and the other at the ankle, force is applied outwards. **For adduction test:** Change hand to the medial side of the knee and give an adduction force. | Positive in injury to the medial structures of the knee like tibial collateral ligament. Positive in injuries to lateral structures of knee like fibular collateral ligament. |
| **Lachman's* test** (Fig. 1.8B) 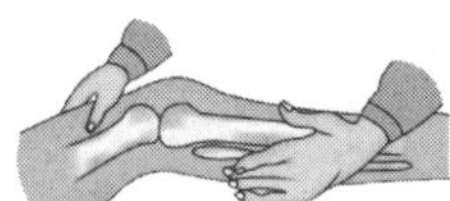 **Fig. 1.8B** | This is an anterior drawer's test done at 20–30° of knee flexion with patient in supine position. | Indicates ACL tear. This test is used in acute injuries of knee to test ACL tear where knee cannot be flexed to 90°. |
| **Anterior Drawer's test** (Fig. 1.8C) 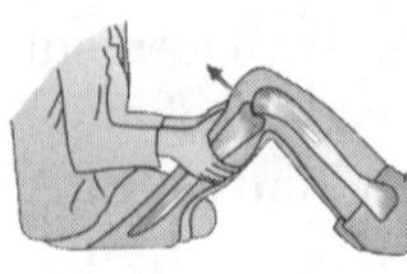 **Fig. 1.8C** | Patient is in supine position. Hip is flexed to 45° and knee to 90°. Examiner sits on the dorsum of the foot and pulls the tibia forwards. The anterior drawer's test is done in 3 positions: a. Foot in neutral position—if positive, it indicates ACL tear, etc. b. Foot in 15° internal rotation—if positive, indicates damage to anterolateral structures. c. Foot in 15° external rotation—if positive, indicates damage to anteromedial structures. | If the tibia shifts anteriorly more than 6–8 mm, then it indicates torn ACL and the test is considered as positive. This should always be compared with the normal knee. |

*Contd...*

**Table 1.1:** Clinical tests to diagnose various knee ligament injuries*(Contd.)*

| | | |
|---|---|---|
| **Posterior Drawer's test** (Fig. 1.8D) 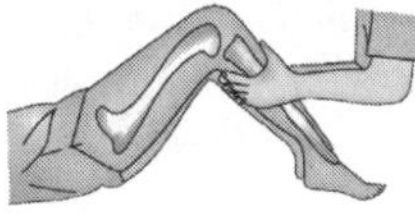 **Fig. 1.8D** | Same as above but tibia is pushed backwards. Positive test is indicated by the movement of the tibia backwards. | Indicates posterior cruciate ligament tear. |
| **Jerk test of Hughston** (Fig. 1.8E) 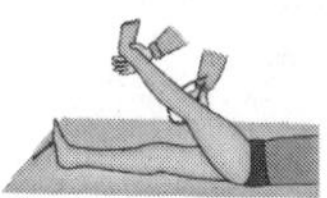 **Fig. 1.8E** | Patient is supine, knee is flexed to 90°. Tibia is internally rotated with a valgus force applied at the knee, it is slowly extended. *Lateral tibial condyle subluxates at 30° and spontaneous relocation occurs as knee extends.* | *Inference* indicates anterior cruciate ligament tear and is more specific than Drawer's test in detecting ACL tear. |
| **Pivot shift test** (Fig. 1.8F) 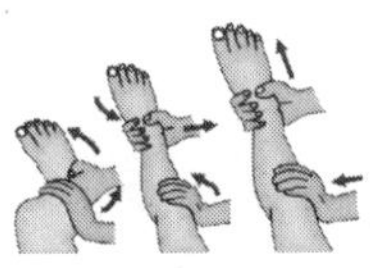 **Fig. 1.8F** | Patient is supine. The knee is extended, with a valgus stress applied on the knee and the tibia is internally rotated. The knee is slowly flexed. Subluxation occurs at 30-40°. | A positive test indicates anterior cruciate ligament tear. |

**Disturbing facts: About ACL tear**

ACL tear → Knee instability → Repeated episodes of instability leads to damage to menisci, cartilage and other ligaments → This ultimately leads to secondary OA knee.

**Clinical tests** (For medical readers)

- *Slocum test:* It is an anterior drawer's test (rotary test) performed with 15° of internal rotation and 30° of external rotation. The former is positive in anterolateral instability and the latter in anteromedial instability.
- *External rotation recurvatum test (posterior sag sign):* When the leg is passively lifted by holding the toes, the knee sags posteriorly indicating injury to PCL and poster lateral structures.
- *Lachman's test* (Fig. 1.9) as already described, this is an anterior drawer's test done at 20–30° of flexion. It has several advantages over 90° flexion anterior drawer's test. The following are some of them:
  - It can be done in the presence of effusion and hence is useful in acute cases when knee cannot be flexed up to 90°.
  - Evokes less pain as full flexion is not required.
  - Hamstrings and torn menisci will not block forward glide easily.
  - More specific for posterolateral fibers of ACL tear.

**Grading of Lachman's test**

- Grade I: End feel appreciation (0–5 mm displacement).
- Grade II: Visible anterior movement of tibia (5-10 mm displacement).
- Grade III: Gross anterior tibial translation (more than 10 mm displacement).

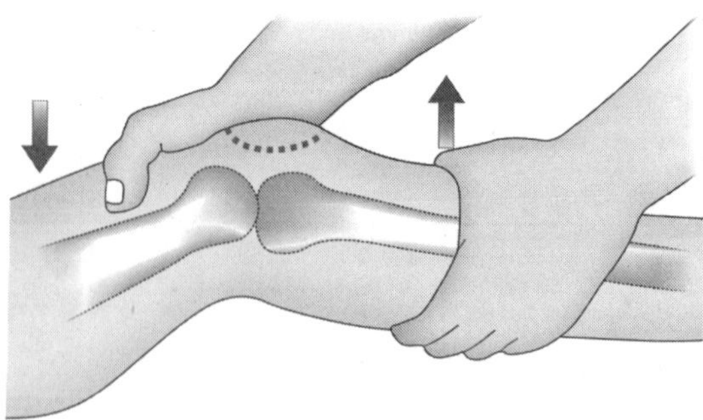

**Fig. 1.9:** Lachman's test

## Investigations in ACL Tear

*Radiograph of the knee:* The views recommended are antero-posterior (AP) view, lateral view, intercondylar notch view, sunrise views, etc. Radiographs are usually normal in ACL tear. Avulsion fracture of tibial spine if present indicates ACL tear.

**Did you know, what a Segund fracture is?**

It is an avulsion fracture of the inferior lateral capsule adjacent to the tibia. If present, it suggests ACL tear.

*MRI:* This is the best diagnostic tool. It is noninvasive and demonstrates the ACL tear with remarkable accuracy. This is the gold standard investigation for ACL tears and has virtually replaced all others.

*KT-1000:* This measuring system documents anteroposterior tibial displacement by tracking the tibial tubercle in rotation to the patella. More than 3 mm anterior displacement at 20 lb predicts an ACL tear with 94 percent accuracy.

## How to manage these injuries? Treatment of ACL Tear

### *Conservative*

This is reserved for Grade I and II tears and consists of rest, long leg casts for 4–6 weeks, NSAIDs, physiotherapy, etc.

### *Surgical*

Surgery is reserved for more severe tears and the techniques vary from primary repair, reinforcements or reconstruction of the ACL ligament depending upon the extent and duration of time.

Arthroscopically assisted ACL reconstruction has been universally advocated due to its superior results.

*Fresh:* Primary repair is indicated in young adults and athletes. Repair is successful if ACL is torn at its femoral or tibial attachments. It is not successful in midposition tears. Failure rate is as high as 50 percent.

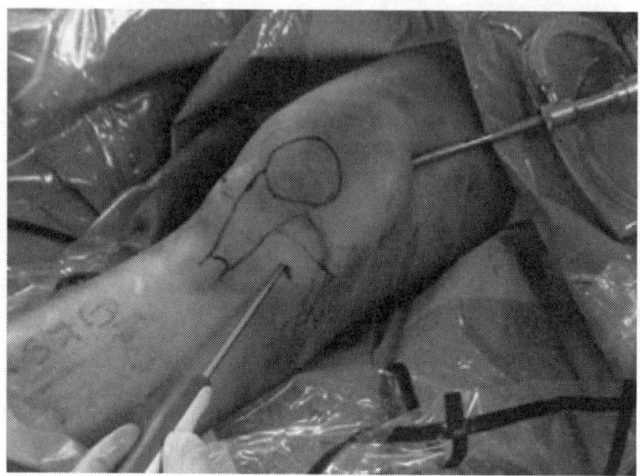

**Fig. 1.10A:** Arthroscopic surgeries are the gold standard for ACL reconstruction

*Old cases*

- Reinforcement of ACL tear should be augmented except when avulsion is with a fragment of bone. Reinforcement could be either intra-articular or extra-articular or both by using iliotibial band, semitendinosus tendon, etc.
- Reconstruction in chronic ACL insufficiency could be either intra-articular or extra-articular replacement by using quadriceps, tendon, patellar tendon (central 1/3) bone patella tendon bone graft (BPTB) (Fig. 1.10B), semitendinosus tendon, gracilis, etc.

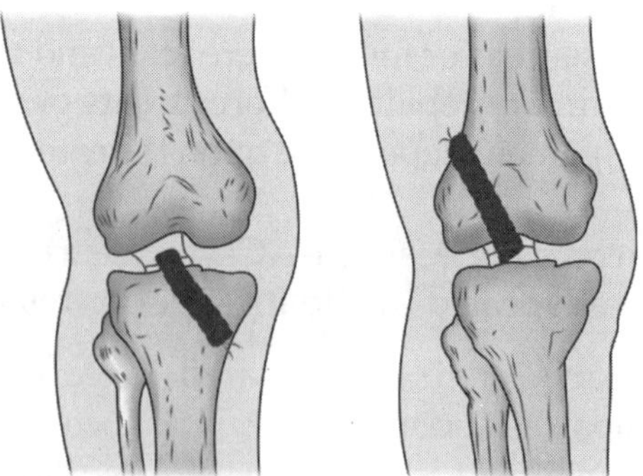

**Fig. 1.10B:** Methods of ACL repair

These autografts are preferred over allograft, which are reserved for:

- Revision ACL reconstruction.
- Rupture of both ACL and PCL.

**Surgical Technique of ACL Reconstruction in a Nutshell**

- Graft harness and preparation
- Notchplasty
- Tibial tunnel placement
- Femoral tunnel placement
- Graft passage

**Remember**

Autografts widely used in reconstruction of ACL tear

- Central 1/3 of patellar tendon (BPTB Graft)
- Semitendinous and gracilis tendons

**Vital points: ACL tear**

- Common in young active people usually athletes may interfere with activity or it may make activity impossible.
- Usually it does not tear in isolation.
- Associated with other ligament injuries.
- May predispose to menisci lesions.
- May predispose to OA changes.

## POSTERIOR CRUCIATE LIGAMENT (PCL) TEAR

It is less common than ACL tear. It is ruptured due to severe rotational injury, dashboard injury or complete dislocation of the knee. Isolated PCL tear is rare and is accompanied with other ligament injuries.

*Note:* PCL tear accounts for 3–4 percent of all knee ligament injuries.

### Clinical Features

The patient complains of pain, swelling and tenderness over the popliteal fossa. Clinically, posterior drawer test and sag sign will be positive (Fig. 1.11).

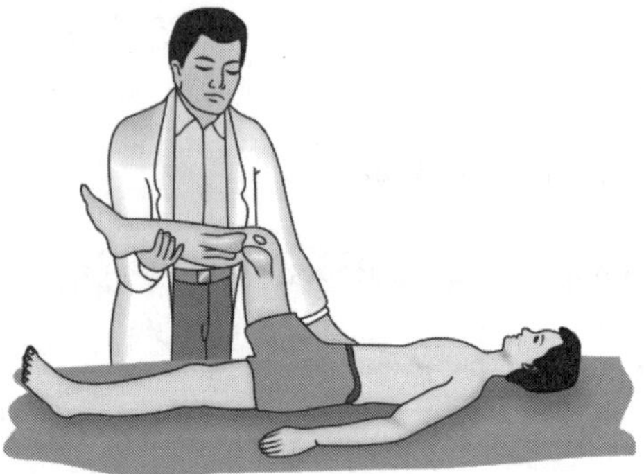

**Fig. 1.11:** Posterior 'sag sign' for PCL tear

**Pearl**

Ninety degrees posterior drawer test is the most important test to diagnose PCL tear.

**Investigations:** These are similar to ACL tear.

**Conservative:** Most of the Grade I and II PCL tears can be treated nonoperatively.

**Surgery:** This is indicated in Grade III injuries with posterior translation > 10 mm. Reconstruction is done by using medial head of gastrocnemius, etc.

Avulsion of the PCL from the femoral or tibial ends is more common unlike in ACL tears. Here reattachment of the avulsed ligament usually gives good results. Reconstruction is reserved for:

- Midsubstance tears.
- Old tears.

**Graft Options for PCL Reconstruction**

- Central one-third of patellar tendon.
- Patella tendon allograft.
- Achilles tendon allograft.
- Semitendinosus or gracilis graft.
- Two-tailed femoral graft is the graft of choice.
- Some prefer anterolateral femoral reconstruction with a tibial inlay grafting.

## COMBINED KNEE LIGAMENT INJURIES

Rupture of the cruciate and collateral ligaments either singly (rare) or in combination (common) makes the knee unstable. Depending upon the combination of injuries, the knee instability could be either one plane, two planes or both (Table 1.2). Table 1.3 depicts the knee instabilities in different planes, the various tests and the structures of the knee injured.

**Table 1.2:** Knee instability in different planes

| | |
|---|---|
| If only medial structures torn | One plane medial instability |
| If only lateral structures torn | One plane lateral instability |
| If ACL and medial structures torn | Two plane anterior and medial instability |
| If ACL and lateral structures torn | Two plane anterior and lateral instability |
| If PCL and medial structures torn | Two plane posterior and medial instability |
| If PCL and lateral structures torn | Two plane posterior and lateral *instability* |

**Combined instabilities of knee**

- If anterior, medial and lateral structures are torn. — Anteromedial and anterolateral instabilities.
- If anterior, posterior cruciates lateral structures are torn. — Anterolateral and posterolateral instabilities.
- If anterior, posterior cruciates and medial structures are torn. — Anteromedial and posteromedial instabilities.

*Anterolateral instability:* This is due to injury of anterolateral structures. Reconstruction is done by using iliotibial band or biceps femoris transfer.

*Posterolateral instability:* This is due to injury to the posterolateral structures. Posterolateral structures repair or reconstruction is recommended.

*Posteromedial instability:* This is due to injury to the posteromedial structures. Repair or reconstruction of posteromedial structures is done.

**At a glance**

**Cruciate injuries**

- ACL commonly tears than PCL (9:1).
- Commonest mechanism for ACL tear is external rotation with abduction of a flexed knee and for PCL tear dashboard injury.
- Rarely tears in isolation.
- Commonly tears in combinations.
- May tear at midsubstance or femoral and tibial attachments.
- ACL tear is a common cause of hemarthroses (70%).
- Lachman's test is useful in acute ACL tear.
- Drawer's test, rotary test, etc. helps in the diagnosis of combination tears.
- Treatment is by three **R's**
  - **R**epair in fresh cases
  - **R**einforce in old lax ligaments
  - **R**econstruct in old torn ligaments
- Predisposes to instability and osteoarthritis changes.

**Collateral injuries**

- Medial collateral injury is more common than lateral.
- Medial collateral injury is due to valgus force.
- Ligament sprain is graded into three degrees.
- Stress tests help in the diagnosis.
- Usually associated with other ligament injuries.
- First and second-degree sprain managed conservatively.
- Third degree sprain needs surgical repair.
- Old tears need reconstruction or distal transfer.

## SEMILUNAR CARTILAGE INJURIES

### Anatomy

The semilunar cartilages are two crescent-shaped plates of fibrocartilage that are placed on the condylar surface of the tibia. They are commonly known as medial and lateral menisci and are unique in that not all species have menisci in their knees and not all joints have menisci (Table 1.4). They are vital for the function of the knee joint (Fig. 1.12). The vascular supply to both the menisci is from the lateral, medial and middle geniculate vessels. The depth of vascular penetration at the periphery is 10–30 percent width of medial meniscus and 10–25 percent width of lateral meniscus. In

**Table 1.3:** Classification of knee instability after performing the various tests mentioned earlier

| **I. One plane instability** | **Tests** | **Structures injured** |
|---|---|---|
| One plane medial → | Abduction stress positive | Tibial collateral ligament + Medial capsule |
| One plane lateral → | Adduction stress positive → | Lateral capsule + Fibular collateral ligament |
| One plane posterior → | Posterior Drawer's test positive → | PCL + Arcuate complex |
| One plane anterior → | Anterior Drawer's test positive → | ACL + Medial and lateral capsular ligament |
| **II. Two plane instability (rotary)** | | |
| Anteromedial → | Slocum's test +ve →<br>Rotary test +ve | ACL + TCL + Posterior oblique ligament + Medial capsular tear. |
| Anterolateral → | Slocum's test +ve →<br>Rotary test +ve | LCL + ACL + Arcuate complex + Lateral capsule. |
| Posteromedial → | Posterior drawer's, reverse pivot shift test, recurvatum test positive. → | TCL + Medial capsule + Posterior oblique ligament + ACL + Posteromedial capsule |
| Posterolateral → | Same as above → | FCL + PCL Arcuate complex + Lateral capsule |
| **III. Combined** | | |
| a. Anterolateral posteromedial → instability: (most common) | Anterior drawer's test positive in → neutral Ext and Int rotation position | Anterior posterior lateral and medial structures injured of the knee |
| b. Anterolateral posterolateral → instability: | External rotation recurvatum test → positive | Anterolateral and posterolateral structures |
| c. Anteromedial and → posteromedial instability: | Knee opens medially →<br>Tibia rotates anteriorly at first and then moves posteriorly | Anteromedial and posteromedial structures |

TCL—tibial collateral ligament, ACL—anterior cruciate ligament, PCL—posterior cruciate ligament, FCL—fibular collateral ligament

**Table 1.4:** Comparative study between medial and lateral meniscus

| | *Features* | *Medial meniscus* | *Lateral meniscus* |
|---|---|---|---|
| 1 | Shape | Semicircular | Circular |
| 2 | Anterior horn | Attached to tibial intercondylar eminence in front of ACL | To intercondylar eminence of tibia lateral to ACL |
| 3 | Posterior horn | Intercondylar area in front of PCL and behind posterior horn of lateral meniscus | To the intercondylar eminence |
| 4 | Outer aspect | Attached to posterior fibres of TCL | Separated from FCL by capsule and popliteus |
| 5. | Mobility | Less mobile | More mobile |

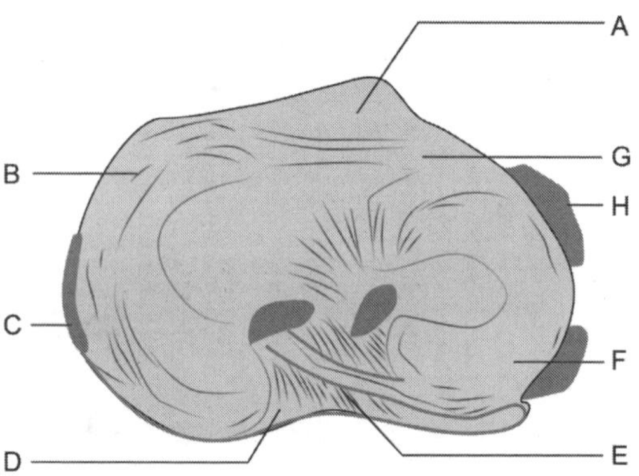


**Fig. 1.12:** Anatomy of two menisci: (A) Tibial tubercle, (B) Lateral meniscus, (C) Fibular collateral ligament, (D) Posterior cruciate ligament, (E) Ligament of Wrisburg, (F) Medial meniscus, (G) Intertransverse ligament, and (H) Medial collateral ligament

cross-section, they appear triangular, the thicker peripheral portion is vascular and heals well and the thin central edge is avascular, receiving nutrition by diffusion and hence heals poorly.

### Functions of the Menisci

- Contributes towards the stability of the knee joint.
- Weight transmission of 40–70 percent of the load across the knee joint.
- Acts as a shock absorber.
- Deepens the tibial condyles on which the femoral condyles roll by increasing the contact area by 40 percent.
- Assists in nutrition of the articular cartilage by distribution of the synovial fluid.
- Helps the knee in locking mechanism.
- Prevents impingement of synovial membrane, capsule, etc.
- Assists and controls gliding and rolling motion of the knee.

## MEDIAL MENISCUS INJURY

Medial meniscus is more commonly injured than the lateral and is usually associated with other ligament injuries of the knee.

### Smillie's Classification

Medial meniscus injury (Figs 1.13A to F) is seen in over 71 percent of the cases. In 5 percent of cases, injury of medial meniscus is bilateral. Lateral meniscus is less commonly injured than the medial meniscus because it is smaller in diameter, thicker in periphery, wide, more mobile, attached to both cruciate ligaments and stabilized posteriorly to the femoral condyle by popliteus.

- *Longitudinal tears* (35%)—in these peripheral attachments tear 10 percent, complete tear 23 percent (bucket handle tear), and segmental tear 2 percent (ant/post).
- *Horizontal tears* (48%)—could be posterior, middle or anterior.
- *Cystic degeneration* (12%).
- *Congenital abnormalities* 5 percent.
- *Regenerative lesions*.

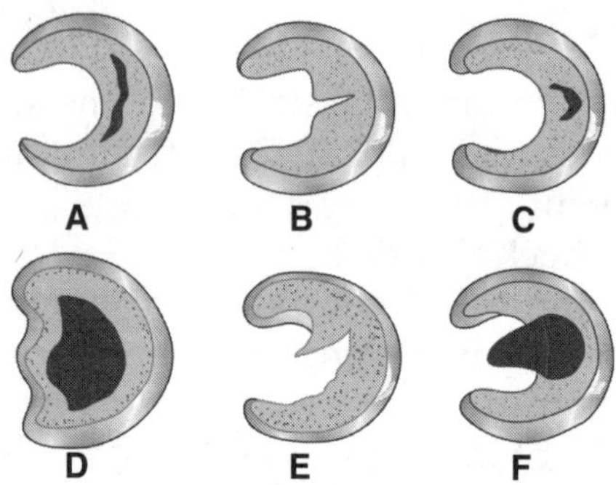


**Figs 1.13A to F:** Different types of meniscal injuries: (A) Longitudinal tear, (B) Radial tear, (C) Horizontal tear, (D) Bucket handle tear, (E) Parrot beak tear, and (F) Segmental tear

## Mechanism of Injury

Mechanism of injury is a rotational force when a flexed knee extends.

- In young, it can occur only when weight is being taken, knee is flexed and there is a twisting strain. Young active athletes are more prone.
- In middle life, fibrosis has decreased the mobility of meniscus and hence tear occurs with less force.

**Predisposing factors:** These could be abnormal menisci shape, abnormal stress due to chronic ligament laxity, etc.

## Clinical Features

The patient with medial meniscus injury presents with pain on the inner aspect of the knee. History of locking is seen in 40 percent of the cases and swelling if present is minimal. There is remarkable recovery after the initial acute attack and there could be periodic complaints pertaining to the knee. One or more clinical signs mentioned in the box can be elicited with careful examination of the knee.

## Investigations

- Radiograph is usually normal. The views recommended are anteroposterior, lateral, intercondylar notch and sunrise views of the patella.

- Arthroscopy helps to identify the torn meniscus (Fig. 1.15).
- Arthrography may reveal the tear. Double contrast arthrography is 95 percent accurate.
- MRI is expensive but useful.

## Differential Diagnosis

Fracture of tibial spine if present may give clue to the possible ACL tear. It also helps to exclude osteochondritis dissecans, osteocartilaginous loose bodies, etc. (Table 1.5).

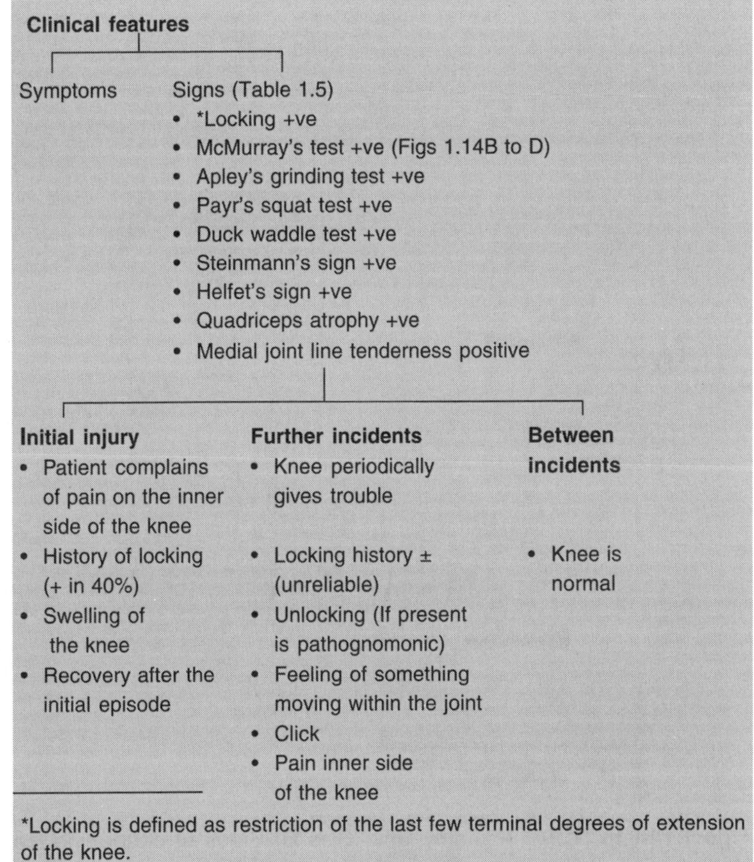

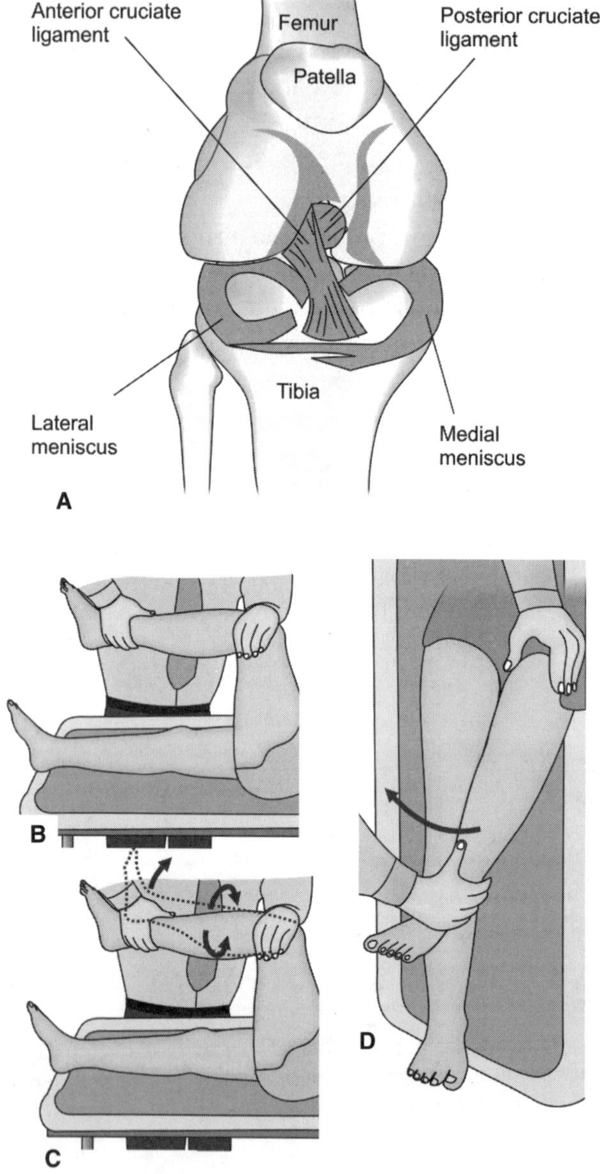


**Figs 1.14A to D:** (A) Anatomy, and (B to D) Steps of performing the McMurray's test (*see* page 26)

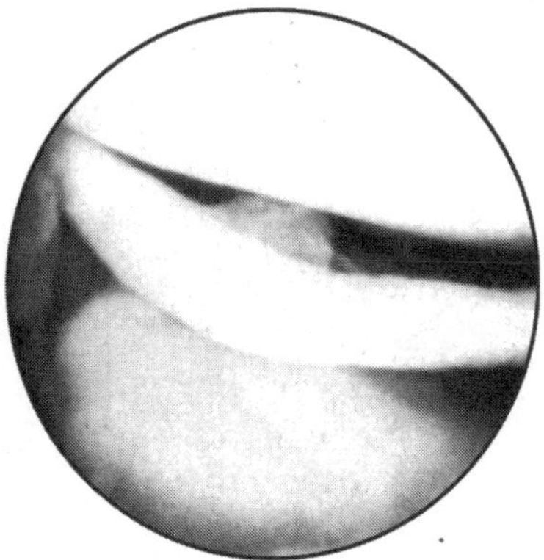

**Fig. 1.15:** Arthroscopic view of a bucket handle tear of medial meniscus injury

**Quick diagnostic points**

**Medial meniscal injuries**

| | |
|---|---|
| Medial joint line tenderness | +ve in 74 percent of cases |
| Apley's grinding test | +ve in 46 percent of cases |
| Painful hyperextension | +ve in 43 percent of cases |
| Steinmann I sign | +ve in 42 percent of cases |
| McMurray's | +ve in 35 percent of cases |

Hence, no one test is diagnostic. That is why multiple tests are required for diagnosis. See for tests (Table 1.5 and Figs 1.16A to G)

## How to manage these injuries? Treatment

*Conservative:* This is indicated in patients soon after injury with no locking and with infrequent attacks of pain and in tears less than 10 mm, partial thickness tears.

### *Measures*

- Abstinence from weight bearing.
- Rest, ice packs, compressive bandage.
- Buck's skin traction.
- Joint aspiration.
- Quadriceps exercises.
- If symptom persists, a cylindrical cast may be considered.

**Table 1.5:** Clinical tests for diagnosis of meniscal injuries

| | | | |
|---|---|---|---|
| Fig. 1.16A | **Joint line tenderness**<br>The medial joint line tenderness is an important clinical sign in detecting medial meniscus injury.<br>It is positive in 74% of the cases (Fig. 1.16A) | 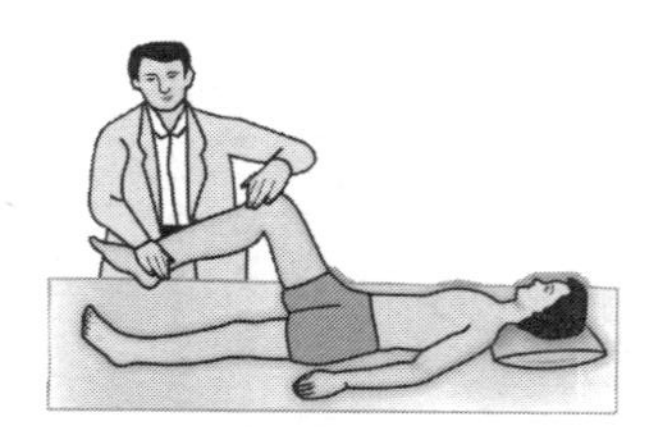 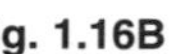<br>Fig. 1.16B | **McMurray's test**<br>Here forced flexion and internal rotation as shown in 1 and external rotation as shown in 2 is done to test the lateral meniscus and the medial meniscus respectively.<br>· A positive McMurray's test requires both pain and clunk to be felt by the examiner's finger on the medial side (Fig. 1.16B). |
| Fig. 1.16C | **Duck Waddle test** (Fig. 1.16C)<br>The patient assumes a squatting position with heels touching the buttock and is asked to perform a duck walk. The patient will be unable to assume full squatting position in medial meniscus injury. This is called as *childress sign* and is a diagnostic test for posterior horn tear of medial meniscus. | 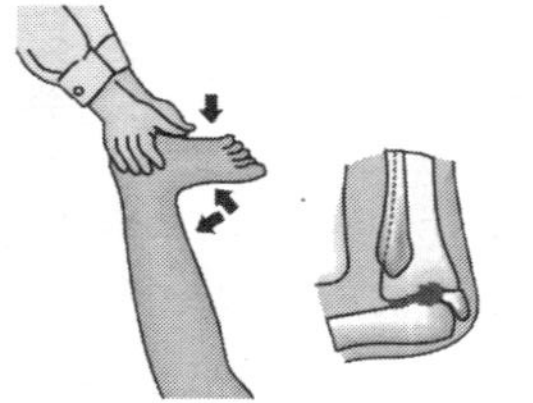<br>Fig. 1.16D | **Apley's compression test** (Fig. 1.16D)<br>The patient is prone, fixing the thigh against the table the examiner presses the foot and leg downward while rotating the tibia (grinding test). Pain noted during axial compression implies a meniscal lesion. |

Contd...

**Table 1.5:** Clinical tests for diagnosis of meniscal injuries *(Contd.)*

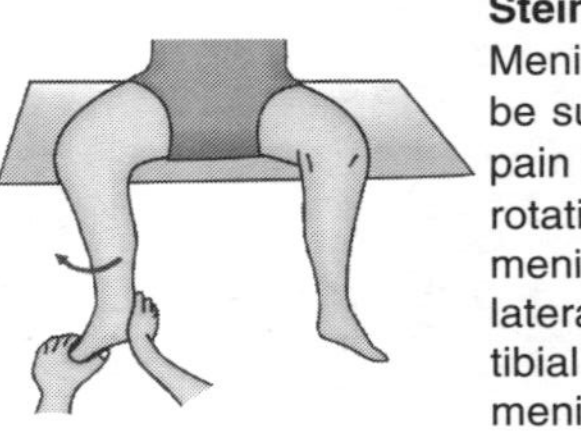

Fig.1.16E

**Steinmann's sign** (Fig. 1.16E)
Meniscal pathology may be suspected if medial pain is elicited on lateral rotation (medial meniscus injury) and lateral pain on medial tibial rotation (lateral meniscal injury).

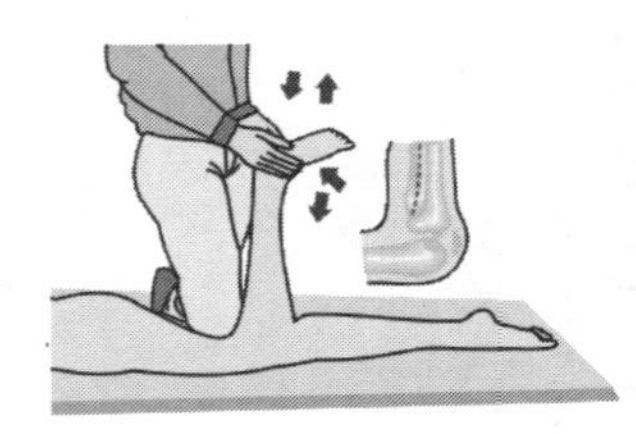

Fig. 1.16F

**Apley's distraction test** (Fig. 1.16F)
The technique is the same as above but here the examiner pulls the foot and leg upward to distract the joint while again rotating the tibia. Pain noted during axial distraction of joint implies a ligamentous lesion.

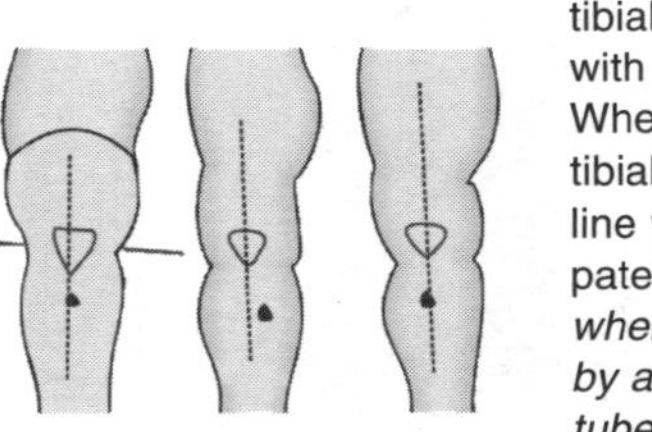

Fig. 1.16G

**Helfet's sign** (Fig. 1.16G)
In normal knee in sitting position tibial tubercle lies in line with midline of the patella. When extended, lateral tibial rotation puts it in line with lateral border of patella. *Positive sign occurs when the rotation is blocked by a torn meniscus and the tubercle remains centred over the patella in extension.*

***Note***

1. *The Apley's test is unique among the meniscus tests because of its ability to distinguish between ligamentous and meniscal lesions.*
2. *Positive meniscus test confirms the suspicion of meniscal lesion. However, negative tests do not rule out a tear with absolute confidence.*
3. *No one test is diagnostic, hence a combination of tests are carried out. With this, the accuracy rate* for *diagnosis raises by 60-95 percent.*
4. *The routine work-up could best include joint line tenderness. McMurray's test and Steinmann's sign.*

*Manipulation under anesthesia:* If joint is locked due to the torn menisci, manipulation under anesthesia is recommended.

### Surgery

*Indications:* Surgery is indicated, if joint cannot be unlocked and if symptoms are recurrent.

### Methods

- *Arthroscopic menisci repair:* This is the treatment of choice of late. Repair is indicated if the tear is > 10 mm or is unstable on probing. Repair is successful in the outer third (red-red zone) edge of the vascular rim (red-white zone) and even in a few avascular zone (white-white zone) (Fig. 1.17A).

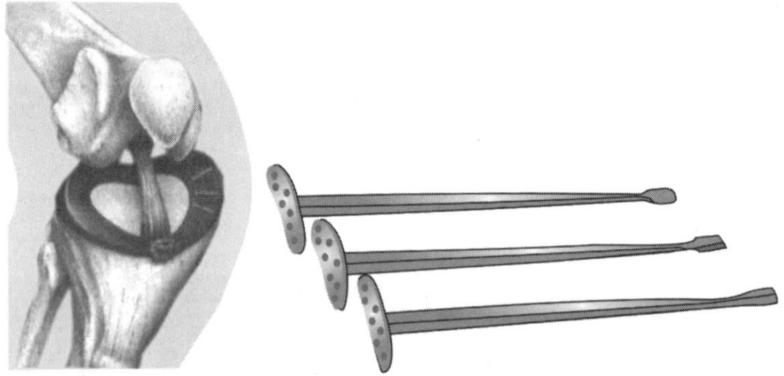

**Fig. 1.17A:** Arthroscopic meniscal repair

**Fig. 1.17B:** Smillie's meniscus knife used for meniscectomy

- *Closed partial meniscectomy* via an arthroscopy is better than total removal of the menisci by open surgery (Fig. 1.17B).
- *Meniscal transplant:* In cases with total menisectomies, cadaver menisci transplant may be considered. However, this is still in the evolving stage.

Complete removal of the menisci incapacitates the knee hence, the emphasis is on conservative surgery than the radical removal.

**Table 1.6:** Differential diagnosis of locking

| *True locking* | *Pseudolocking* |
|---|---|
| 1. Loose bodies | 1. Ligament injuries |
| 2. Recurrent dislocation of patella | 2. Chondromalaciae patella |
| 3. Fracture of tibial spine | |
| 4. Meniscal injuries | |

**Treatment facts: Menisci injuries**

- Nothing like normal meniscus.
- If minor lesion and asymptomatic better leave it alone.
- Partial meniscectomy better than total.
- Resuturing in appropriate locations.
- Earlier it was said, when in doubt remove, now the concept is when in doubt, observe do not treat.

*Note:* How important are menisci to the knee?

*Consider the following facts:*
Partial meniscectomy increases stress by 50–60 percent. Total meniscectomy increases stress by 200–235 percent.
*Menisci repair may normalize the stress.*

## FRACTURE OF PATELLA

Patella is the largest sesamoid bone in the body. The clinical picture of a patellar fracture is determined by a combination of definite and equivocal signs.

**Functions of Patella**

- Increases the mechanical advantage of quadriceps tendon by increasing the efficiency of extensor mechanism by as much as 50 percent due to increased lever arm.
- To aid in the nourishment of articular cartilage.
- To protect the femoral condyles from injury.
- Acts as a hydraulic brake.

**Incidence** is around 1 percent of all skeletal fractures.

## Mechanism of Injury

*Direct trauma:* This is due to dashboard injuries and due to direct fall over the patella (Fig. 1.18). They usually cause comminuted fractures, and are the common causes.

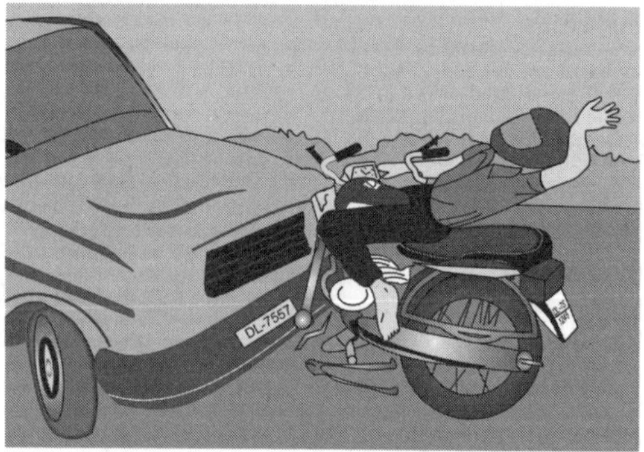


**Fig. 1.18:** Direct injuries due to road traffic accidents (RTAs) are a common cause of patellar fractures

> **Incriminating facts**
>
> Subcutaneous location of patella makes it more vulnerable for direct injures.

*Indirect trauma (Quadriceps contraction):* Sudden forceful contraction of the quadriceps as in sports person and athletes can cause patellar fractures. Here the fracture is usually transverse and sometimes avulsion fractures of the proximal or distal poles may be seen.

*Age:* Common in 20–50 years age group.

*Male: Female* = 2: 1.

## Classification (Figs 1.19A to D)

- Undisplaced:
  - Transverse fracture—these account for nearly 50–80 percent of cases. About 80 percent occur in the middle-third.

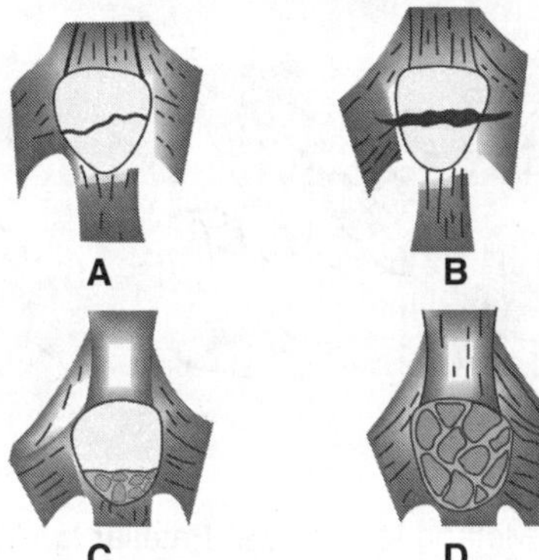


**Figs 1.19A to D:** Types of patellar fractures: (A) Undisplaced fracture, (B) Transverse fracture, (C) Distal pole fracture, and (D) Comminuted fracture

- Stellate fracture.
- Vertical fracture.

- Displaced: If displacement is > 3 mm and if articular incongruity > 2 mm
  - Transverse—involving upper or lower poles (50–85%).
  - Oblique fracture.
  - Vertical fracture (12–27%).
  - Comminuted fracture (30–35%).
  - Polar—could be proximal or distal.
  - Osteochondral fractures.

## Clinical Features

The patient gives history of trauma following which there is pain and swelling at the knee joint. The patient is unable to extend the knee and both the active and passive movements are restricted. On examination, there could be a palpable gap, tenderness, signs of effusion and a positive patellar tap (Figs 1.20A and B).

## Investigations

- Radiograph of the knee joint consists of AP view, lateral view, intercondylar notch view (Fig. 1.21) and skyline or

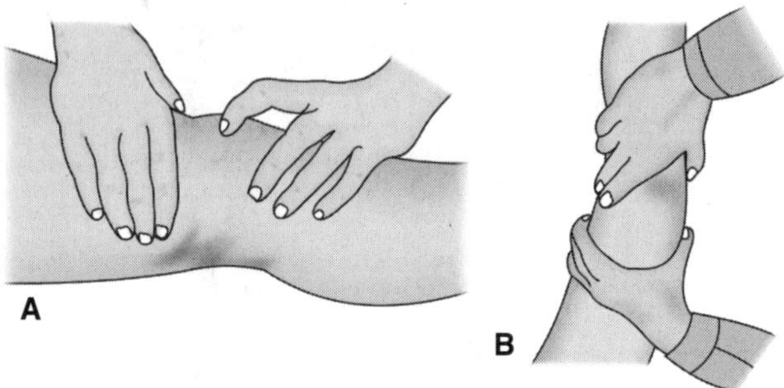


**Figs 1.20A and B:** Method to elicit: (A) Patellar tap, and (B) Fluctuation test

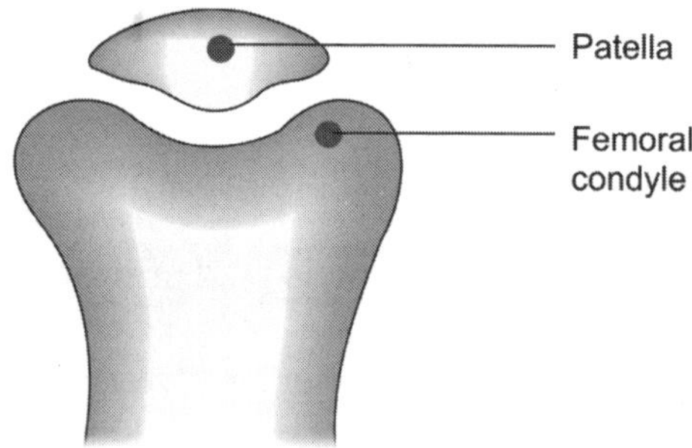


**Fig. 1.21:** Intercondylar notch view of patella

axial view (Fig. 1.22) to rule out undisplaced vertical fracture.

- CT scan, bone scan and tomography are other useful investigations.

*Note:* Bipartite patella and osteochondral fractures cause confusion in the diagnosis (Figs 1.23A and B).

**Mystifying facts**

- Do you know which patellar fractures are difficult to diagnose clinically? Well, it is the thin vertical fracture of the patella which has a very few clinical signs and symptoms.

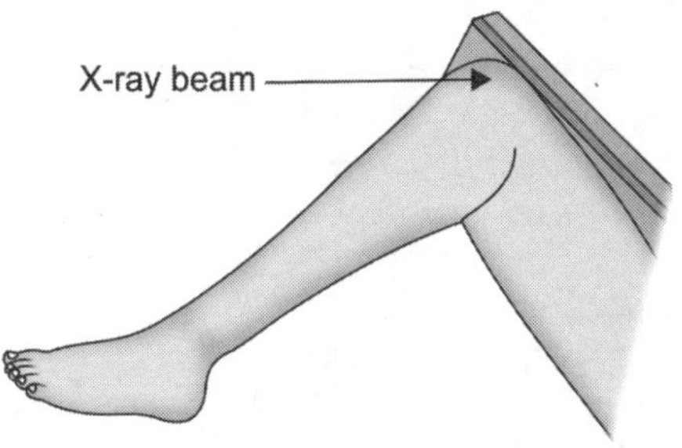


**Fig. 1.22:** Axial view of the knee

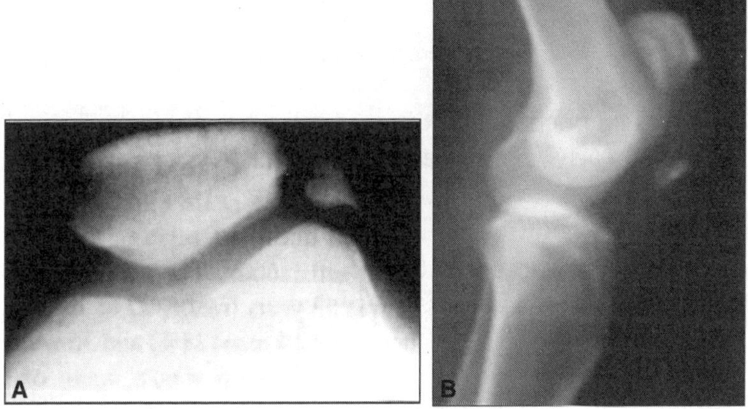


**Figs 1.23A and B:** Radiograph showing bipartite patella: (A) Diagnostic pitfall, and (B) Fracture patellar pole

## Management

### *Undisplaced Fracture*

Nonoperative treatment will produce good results in undisplaced fracture and if displacement is less than 1–2 mm and in intact extensor mechanism and minimal articular step-off (< 1–2 mm) and the methods include compression bandage, ice applications, aspiration of hemarthrosis, cylindrical cast in extension (Fig. 1.24), or long leg cast for

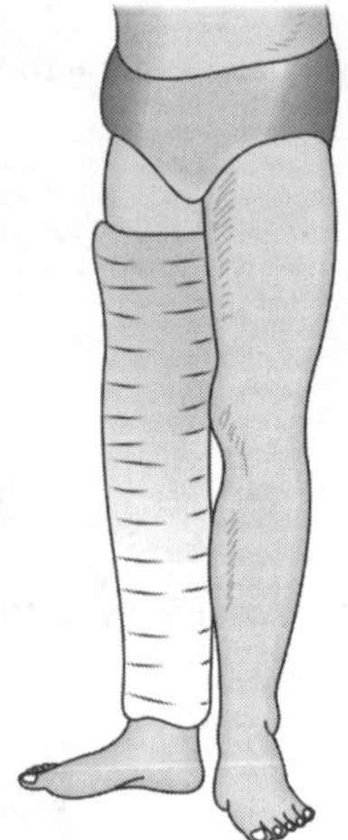

**Fig. 1.24:** Cylindrical cast

4–6 weeks. Functional cast brace is also effective. The patient is advised early weight bearing and quadriceps exercises.

### *Displaced Fracture*

In this variety, surgery is the treatment of choice. Surgery is performed as early as possible preferably within 7 days.

## Surgical Methods

*Open reduction and internal fixation:* This is indicated in transverse fractures of the patella. Internal fixation is done either by the circumferential wiring or by tension band wiring (*see* box). The other methods are Pyrford technique of circumferential wiring and a second tension band wiring through the tendon provide better fixation. Lotke longitudinal anterior band (LAB) wiring is another method with good results.

*Patellectomy:* This could be either partial (for smaller distal or proximal pole fracture) or complete (for comminuted fractures). The emphasis is now on preserving as much patella as possible.

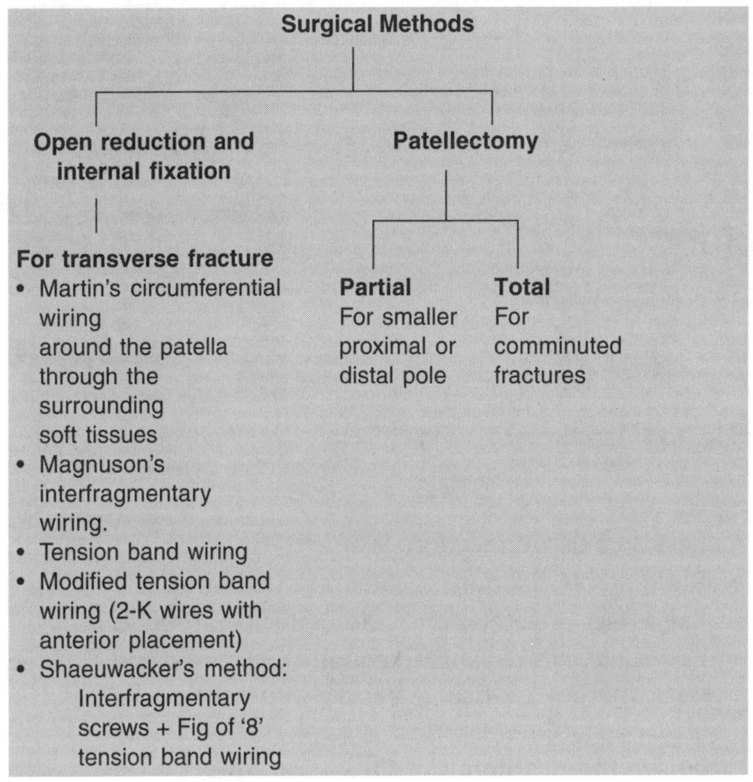


### Wiring of the fracture from front called Anterior Tension Band Wiring (ATBW)

ATBW (Figs 1.25 and 1.26) though a popular method of stabilization of mainly transverse patellar fractures, K-wires, offer the following problems:

- Migration of K-wire up and down.
- Breakage/protrusion.
- Bursa formation.

### Cannulated Screws Fixation

These problems are overcome if TBW is done with two cannulated screws instead of 2 K-wires. Other advantages are:

- Early mobilization of the knee.

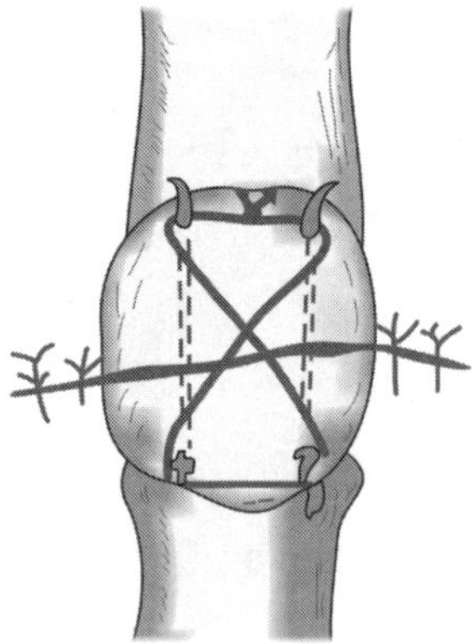

Fig. 1.25: Tension band wiring

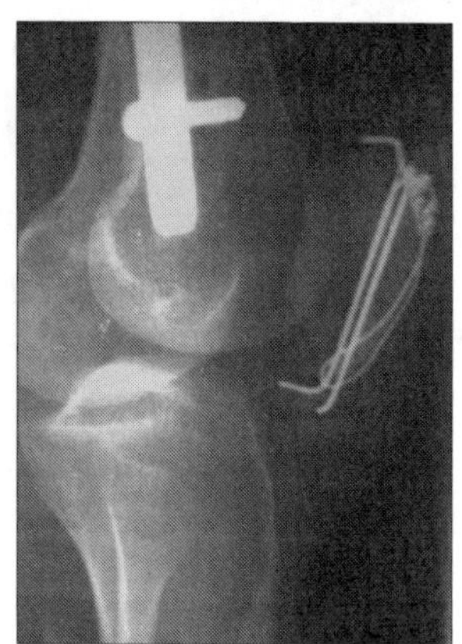

Fig. 1.26: Radiograph showing TBW fracture patella

- Less soft tissue reaction.
- Rigid stable fixation in osteoporotic bones.
- Lag effect of screws provide better compression.
- Destructive forces shared equally by screws, and circlage wire, thereby reducing chances of breakage.

## What are the problems of these fractures? Complications

*Postoperative Complications*

- Early fracture dehiscence,
- Postoperative infection,
- Refracture (1–5%),
- Avascular necrosis (25% incidence in proximal pole) are some of the common postoperative complications.

*Delayed Complications*

- Knee stiffness,
- Osteoarthritis of the patellofemoral joint,
- Knee joint extensor lag,
- Delayed union,

- Nonunion,
- Loss of knee motion, etc.

*What are the Disadvantages of Patellectomy*

- Strength of quadriceps returns slowly although knee motion is regained quite fast.
- Obvious atrophy of the quadriceps muscle persists for months and often permanently.
- Protection of the knee by the patella is lost.
- Pathological ossification may develop where the patella is excised.

**Extensor lag (This is a peculiar complication of patella fractures)**

This is inability of the patient to perform the last 10° of extension (Fig. 1.27). About 80 percent of quadriceps strength is required to bring about the last 20° of extension. After patellectomy, due to the decreased lever arm, the efficiency of quadriceps is reduced and the patient will be unable to bring about the terminal extension of the knee. Thus, an attempt is made to save as much of patella as possible, all of the patella or at least the proximal or distal half, if practical to preserve the quadriceps efficiency.

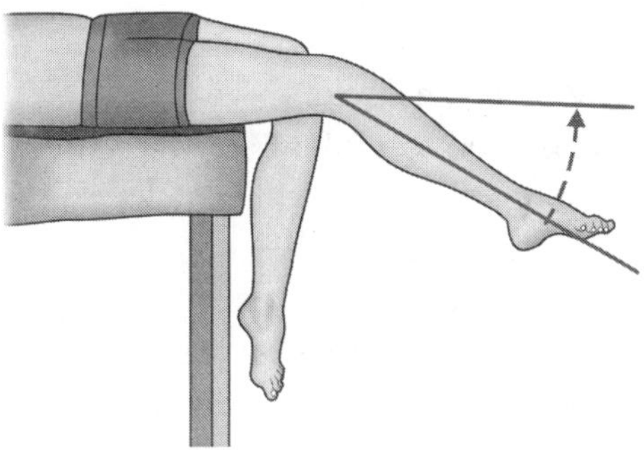

**Fig. 1.27:** Extensor lag

**Disturbing facts**

Do you know the common sequelae of patellar fractures?
- Patellofemoral arthritis.
- Instability of the knee.
- Decreased ROM of the knee.
- Difficulty with stairs, downhill walking and kneeling.

**What is new in the treatment of patellar fractures?**
Arthroscopically assisted percutaneous screw fixation for displaced patellar fracture is being tried with varied success.

## INJURY TO THE EXTENSOR APPARATUS OF KNEE

The extensor apparatus of the knee is comprised of the following six structures:

- The quadriceps muscle with a group of six extensor muscles and the quadriceps femoris tendon.
- Patella.
- Ligamentum patellae (patellofemoral and patellotibial ligaments).
- Patellar bursae and the fat pads.
- Capsule and synovial membrane.

*Note:* The quadriceps muscle consists of rectus femoris, vastus medialis, lateralis intemedius, articularis genu and ligamentum patellae.

## QUADRICEPS STRAIN

### Causes

- Direct blow to the muscle.
- Indirect forces due to violent sudden contractions.

### Sites

- Rectus femoris is the most commonly injured muscle.
- This is followed by vastus medialis, lateralis and intermedius.
- Avulsion may occur at the upper pole of patella or tibial tubercle and rarely through the patella.

## Symptoms

- In rectus femoris injury, the patient complains of pain during hip flexion and knee extension as this muscle is known to act on both these joints. Tenderness is present at the site of injury.
- In grade III sprain a gap may be felt at the site of rupture and ambulation is difficult.
- In injuries to the vastus medialis, intermedius and lateralis the patient may complain of pain and limp, terminal stage of flexion and resisted knee flexion is extremely painful.

## Treatment

In general, grade I and grade II injuries can be managed conservatively, while grade III injury may require surgical suturing in the event of complete rupture and loss of function (Fig. 1.28).

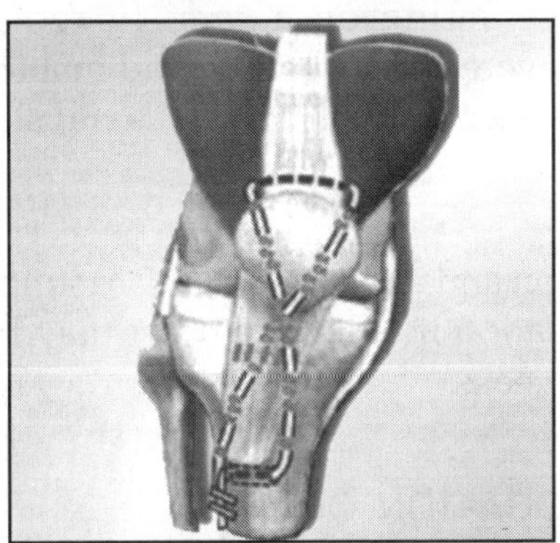

**Fig.1.28:** Reconstruction of extensor mechanism

### *Treatment Methods*

*Grade I and II Strain*

- Ice therapy and ice packs.
- Compression bandaging (Jones).
- Limb elevation.
- Mild isometric exercises.

- Relaxed passive knee movements.
- To improve the strength and mobility of the knee joint, active and active-assisted knee exercises are begun.
- Progressive resistive exercises to increase the endurance of the knee muscles.
- Gradual weight bearing with assistive devices. The patient should be functionally independent by 6 weeks.

*Grade III Strain*

- Quadriceps exercises are begun by 5-6 days.
- Self-assisted SLR.
- By 2nd or 3rd day's nonweight-bearing and partial weight bearing by 3 weeks, full weight bearing by 6 weeks.
- For extensor lag, electrical stimulation helps.
- Rest of the measures is the same as mentioned above.

## ACUTE DISLOCATION OF PATELLA

Lateral dislocations of patella are very common and are due to lateral force acting on a semi-flexed knee. Patient complains of severe pain, swelling and inability to bend the knee. Patella is seen and felt on the lateral side.

### Treatment

Closed reduction and above knee POP casting is done under GA. Immobilization in a long leg cast may be required for a period of 4 weeks.

## ACUTE DISLOCATION OF KNEE

This is an uncommon injury and is due to severe violence as in RTA, fall, etc. It is usually associated with injuries to collateral cruciates and meniscus. Patella may also be fractured or dislocated.

### Treatment

**Conservative:** An attempt may be made for closed reduction under GA. An above knee POP cast is applied for 12 weeks.

**What are the management options? Treatment**

**Conservative Methods:** An attempt may be made for closed reduction under GA. An above knee POP cast is applied for 12 weeks.

**Surgery:** Open reduction may be required if the closed reduction fails or if there is extensive ligament injuries, which may require repair, reconstruction or both. Knee is immobilized in above knee POP cast for 12 weeks.

## ANKLE INJURIES

Pott described ankle injuries for the first time in 1768.

**Interesting 'Incidence facts' about ankle fractures**

- More commonly in elderly women.
- About 2/3 are isolated malleolar fracture.
- About 1/4 are bimalleolar fracture.
- Trimalleolar fracture seen only in 7 percent.
- Open fracture 2 percent.

### Mechanism of Injury

Ankles are usually injured due to low injury rotational forces due to:

- Twisting injury while walking, running, sports, athletes, etc. are the most common mode of ankle injuries (Figs 1.29 and 1.30).
- Fall from a height: Ankle injuries are indirect injuries here brought about by the displacing talus.

### Classification

Ankle injuries are classified after the mechanism causing them. Hence, it is of paramount importance to understand the movement of the ankle to comprehend the classification. What complicates the issue is the practice of using more than one term to describe the same motion.

There are six movements of the ankle and the hind foot. Plantar flexion and dorsiflexion are the up and down movements of the foot. Movement causing the toes to point

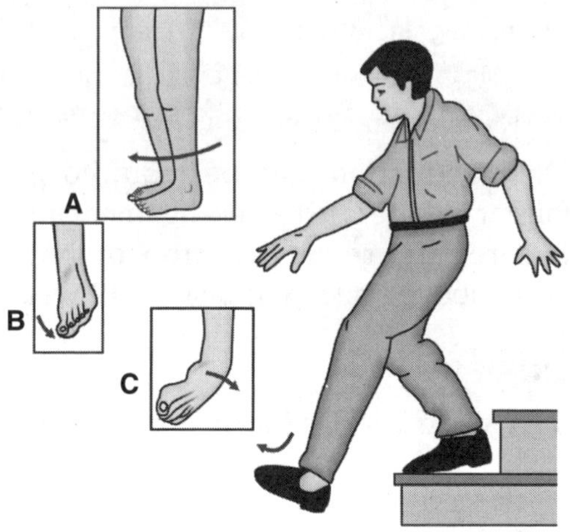


**Figs 1.29A to C:** Common mechanism of ankle injuries: (A) External rotation force, (B) Abduction force, (C) Adduction force. Inversion injury while getting down the stairs is a common mode of ankle injury

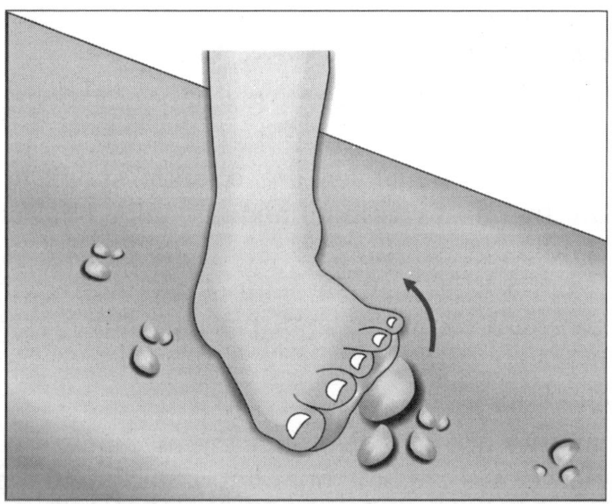

**Fig. 1.30:** Eversion mechanism of ankle injury

inwards is called internal rotation and movement causing the toes to point outwards is called external rotation. Supination is the movement, which raises the medial aspect of the foot and the heel off the ground. In pronation, the motion is to bring the lateral aspect of the foot and the heel from the ground. In adduction, the hind foot is moved towards the midline and in abduction is moved laterally. Pure vertical loading position as in landing, jumping, falling, etc. will cause Pylon fracture by the driving of the talus into the tibia.

### *Lauge Hansen's Classification*

Four major types are described. The mechanism of injury could be adduction force, abduction force or external rotation force. The foot could be in supination or pronation (Figs 1.31A to E). The first word refers to the position of the foot at the time of injury and the second to the direction of injuring force.

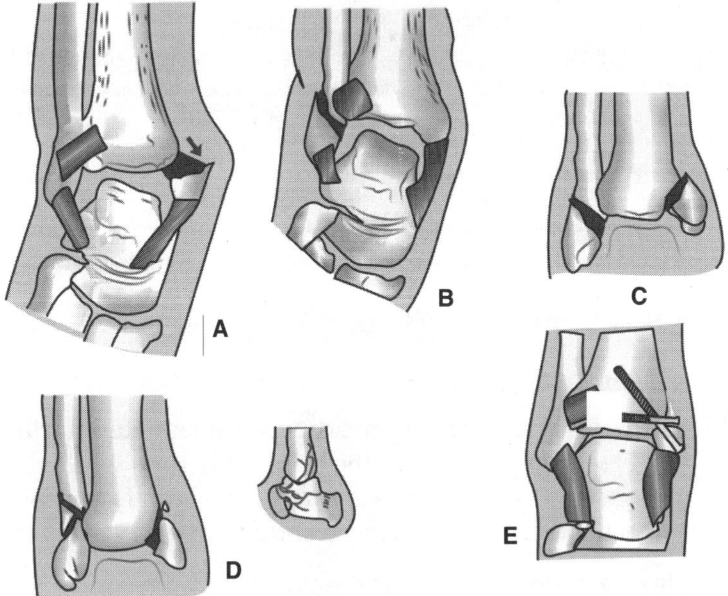


**Figs 1.31A to E:** Lauge Hansen's classification: (A) Supination adduction, (B) Supination eversion, (C) Pronation abduction, (D) Pronation external rotation, (E) Fracture fixed with malleolar screws

**Supination adduction**

Stage I : Transverse fracture of lateral malleolus or tear of lateral collateral ligament.
Stage II : Stage I + fracture of medial malleolus.

**Supination eversion**

Stage I : Rupture of anterioinferior tibiofibular ligament.
Stage II : Stage I + spiral oblique fracture of the lateral malleolus.
Stage III : Stage II + posterior lip of fracture of tibia (posterior malleolar fracture).
Stage IV : Stage III + fracture medial malleolus or tear of deltoid ligament.

**Pronation abduction**

Stage I : Fracture medial malleolus or tear of deltoid ligament.
Stage II : Stage I + rupture of anteroinferior tibiofibular ligament and posteroinferior tibiofibular ligament with fracture posterior lip of tibia.
Stage III : Stage II + oblique supramalleolar fracture of the fibula.

**Pronation-external rotation**

Stage I : Fracture medial malleolus or tear of deltoid ligament
Stage II : Stage I + tear of anteroinferior tibiofibular and interosseous ligament.
Stage III : Stage II + tear of interosseous membrane and spiral fracture of the fibula.
Stage IV : Stage III + fracture of posterior lip of tibia due to ligamentous avulsion by posteroinferior and inferior and transverse tibiofibular ligament.

*Note:* About 75 percent of the cases fall into the first two groups.

### *Denis Weber Classification*

This is the other classification proposed for ankle injuries and it is based on the level of the fibular fracture, while the Lauge Hansen's system is based on experimentally verified injury mechanism like adduction, abduction, etc.

### *AO Classification of Malleolar Fractures*

*Type A:* Infrasyndesmotic (Fracture of fibula below the syndesmosis)

Type A1: Isolated

Type A2: With medial mallelous fracture

Type A3: With posteromedial fracture.

*Type B:* Transsyndesmotic (Fracture of fibula at syndesmosis level).

Type B1: Isolated.

Type B2: With medial lesion (Mallelor or ligament injury).

Type B3: With medial lesion and posterolateral tibial fracture.

*Type C:* Suprasyndesmotic (Fracture of fibula above the sydesmosis).

Type C1: Simple diaphyseal fracture of fibula.

Type C2: Complex diaphyseal fracture of fibula.

Type C3: Proximal fracture of fibula.

## Clinical Features

The patient usually gives history of inversion injury, following which there is pain, swelling, deformity of the ankle. Movements are decreased, Drawer's test, inversion and eversion stress tests may be positive. Note the color and condition of the skin. Examine the entire leg.

## Investigations

Anteroposterior, lateral and mortise non-weight bearing views of the ankle are recommended in the radiographs (Figs 1.32A and B). CT scan, MRI and arthroscopy evaluation is extremely helpful.

## Radiographic Parameters of the Normal Ankle

- Talocrural angle—83° ± 4°.
- Medial clear space 4 mm.
- Tibiofibular clear space < 6 mm.
- Subchondral bone line between the distal tibia and medial surface of lateral malleolus should be continuous.

*Note:* All these parameters are best studied in Mortise views.

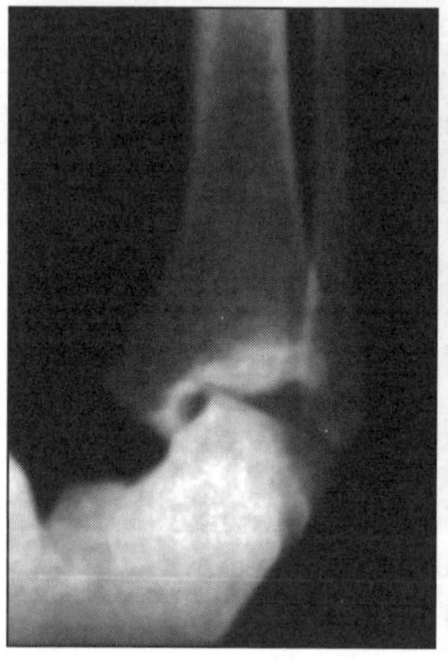

Fig. 1.32A: Radiograph showing inversion injury of ankle

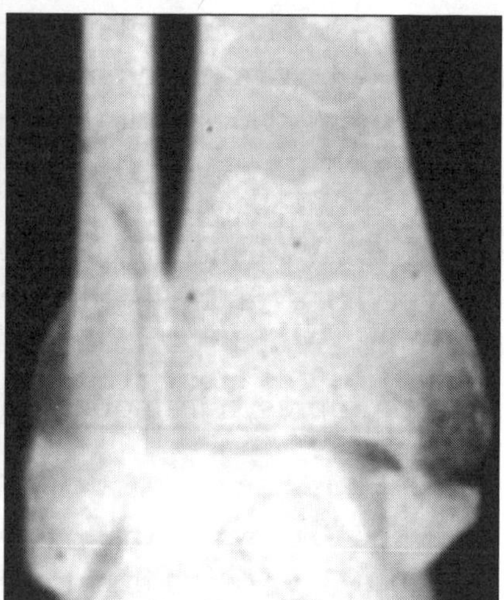

Fig. 1.32B: Radiograph showing bimalleolar ankle fracture

## MALLEOLAR FRACTURES

### How to manage these injuries? Treatment

*Goals*

- Anatomical positioning of the talus beneath the tibia.
- To obtain a joint line that is parallel to the ground.
- Smooth articular surface.

If these three things are not achieved, post-traumatic osteoarthritis results.

*Stable injuries:* No reduction is required, immobilization with only plaster splints till the swelling decreases and then a below knee plaster cast is applied with foot in neutral position.

*Unstable injuries:* Require reduction and immobilization in plaster casts. The commonly encountered unstable injuries are:

- *Fracture due to external rotation:* This is more common and can be managed both by conservative and operative methods.

- *Conservative method:* This consists of reversal of the injuring forces by closed reduction and a below knee plaster cast application (Fig. 1.33). A walking cast is applied after a period of one month.
- *Surgical method:* In this, both the malleoli are fixed, first the lateral malleolus is fixed with pin or screws and later the medial malleolar fracture is fixed with a single screw perpendicular to the fracture line. Below knee splint is given initially and later a cast is applied.

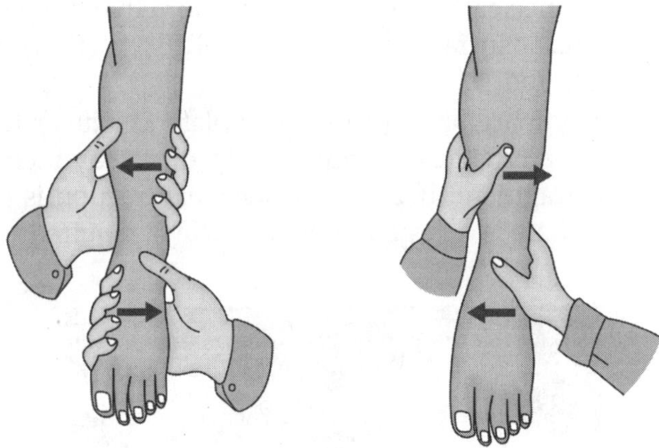

**Fig. 1.33:** Methods of closed reduction of ankle fractures

- *Fracture primarily due to abduction:* These are less common than the fractures due to external rotation. Nevertheless, the principles of the treatment remain the same. Adduction force is required to bring about reduction and if closed reduction fails, open reduction is preferred. During the open reduction, both the malleoli are fixed.
- *Fracture primarily due to adduction:* Unlike external rotation and abduction, adduction violence is more frequently an isolated event. Wedging of small-comminuted fragments into the fracture line often prevents closed reduction, so that open reduction and internal fixation (ORIF) is required more frequently.

Medial malleolus is approached first, since it is more unstable, and the fracture is fixed with two screws, one at right angle to the tibial cortex and another at right angle to the fracture line (Fig. 1.34). Lateral fibular fracture is stabilized with plate and screws.

- *Fracture resulting from primarily vertical compression:* This may be isolated or associated with other forces described above. The anterior and posterior tibial plafond margins are fractured. Two types are described:
  - Posterior marginal fracture for undisplaced fracture, below knee cast is sufficient. For more than 25 percent of articular surface involvement, ORIF with two screws is preferred.
  - Anterior marginal fracture (tibial plafond injury): It may include a crush of the anterior lip or it may include a major fragment. If crushed, calcaneal traction is given and if there is a large fragment, ORIF is required.

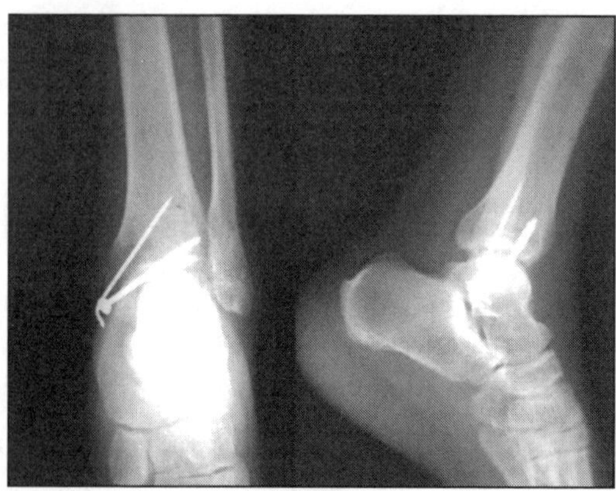

**Fig. 1.34:** Malleolar fixation with screws and K-wire

## TRIMALLEOLAR FRACTURE (COTTON FRACTURE)

This is a difficult injury complex to treat. The salient features about this fracture are:

- It is due to abduction and external rotation injury.

**In a nutshell the fixation techniques for medial malleolar fractures**

- Large fragment fracture — Single lag screw.
- Small fragment fracture — Combination of 4 mm lag screws and a K-wire.
- Low transverse fracture — Tension band wiring or vertical countersunk 4 mm lag screw.

**In a nutshell the fixation techniques for lateral malleolar fractures**

- For fibular fractures: One third semitubular 3.5 mm plate and screws or multiple 3.5 mm lag screws.
- Long oblique fracture: Two lag screws.
- Low transverse fracture: Single 4.5 mm malleolar screw.
- Both Malleoli: Tension band wiring for lateral malleolar fracture and 4 mm lag screw for associated medial mallelor fracture.

**What are problems and Complications of Ankle Fractures?**

Complications of ankle fractures include

- Post-traumatic arthritis,
- Reflex sympathetic dystrophy,
- Neurovascular injury (injury to posterior tibial vessels and nerve),
- Nonunion (due to soft tissue interposition),
- Malunion, etc.

- There is fracture of the medial, lateral and postero-malleolus.
- For plain X-ray 50° external rotation view is preferred.
- It more often requires open reduction and internal fixation.
- If the posterior malleolar fragment is less than 25 percent of the articular surface, then reduction is automatically achieved when the fibular fracture is fixed.
- However, if it is more than 25–30 percent of the articular surface, then it needs to be reduced and fixed internally.
- The results of fixation are usually inferior to that of bimalleolar fixations.

## ANKLE SPRAINS

These are common injury in sports. If improperly treated, it may result in chronic laxity, pain or delayed recovery.

**Quick facts: Involvement of various structures in ankle sprain**

- Complete rupture of the anterior tibiotibular ligament (ATFL) 65 percent.
- Both ATFL and calcaneofibular ligament 20 percent.
- Antero inferior tibiofibular ligament (high ankle sprain) 10 percent.
- Deltoid ligament 3 percent.

## LATERAL LIGAMENT SPRAIN

This is the most common musculoskeletal injury with an incidence of 1/10,000/day. In 85 percent of cases, it is due to inversion of supinated plantar flexed foot. The lateral ligament commonly injured is anterior talofibular ligament followed by calcaneofibular ligament. The posterior talofibular ligament is rarely sprained (Fig. 1.35).

*Note:* Lateral ankle sprain is the most common soft tissue limb injury and < 15 percent actually show a significant fracture.

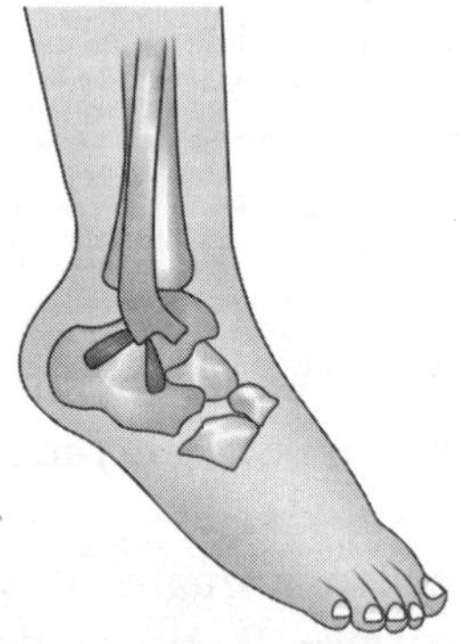

**Fig. 1.35:** Lateral ligament sprain (due to adduction injury)

### Clinical Features

The patient complains of pain, swelling and tenderness over the affected ligament (Fig. 1.36). Anterior drawer test is positive and it is performed by stabilizing distal tibia with one hand, then grasps the posterior heel with the opposite hand and applies anterior force. If the displacement of talus is more than 8 mm anterior, it suggests laxity of the anterior talofibular ligament. Next, the talar tilt test is performed, if the tilt is more than 5°, it suggests laxity of anterior talofibular and calcaneofibular ligaments.

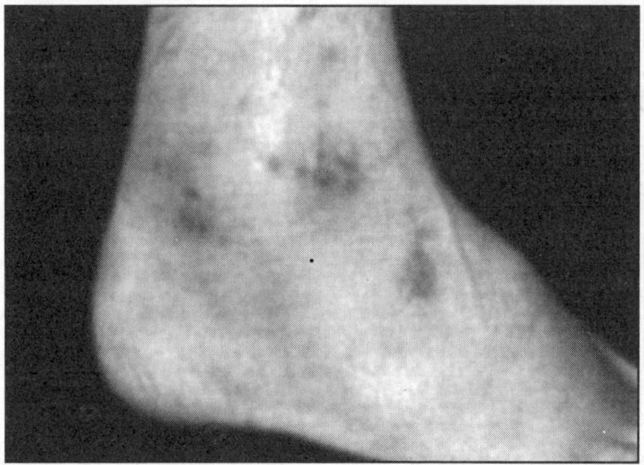

**Fig. 1.36:** Clinical photograph of ankle sprain

## Investigations are a must during ankle sprain?

## Radiograph of the Ankle

Different views like the anteroposterior,lateral and oblique plain X-rays of the ankle are studied. If the talar tilt of the injured ankle is 10° greater than the uninjured ankle, it is considered as significant.

**Vital facts: Ottawa Rules** (Fig. 1.37)

X-rays are required in ankle sprains if:

- There is bony tenderness in the posterior half of lower end of tibia and fibula.
- Tenderness over the fifth metatarsal and navicular bones.
- Inability to bear weight immediately or after 10 days after injury.

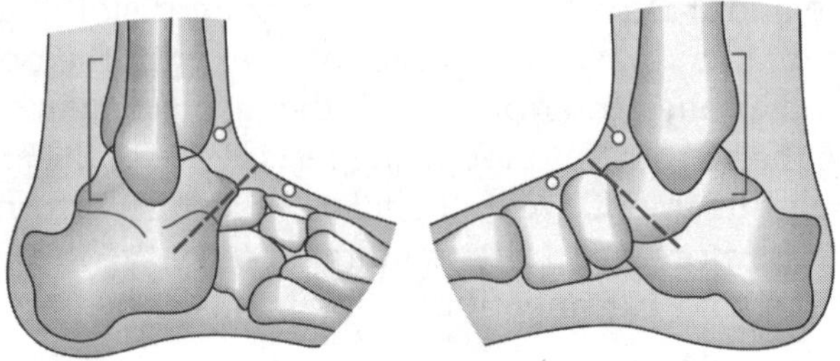

Fig. 1.37: Ankle injuries Ottawa rules

## Grading of Ankle Sprains

*Grade I* : No laxity, minimal pain and mild swelling.

*Grade II* : Mild to moderate laxity, soft tissue swelling, anterior drawer and talar tilt is slightly positive.

*Grade III* : Severe swelling and pain, the anterior drawer and talar tilt tests are highly positive.

## Treatment

*Grade I sprain* : Ice therapy, compression bandage, foot and elevation, ankle strap nonsteroidal anti-inflammatory drugs (NSAIDs), crutch walking, etc. are the recommended treatment (Figs 1.38 and 1.39).

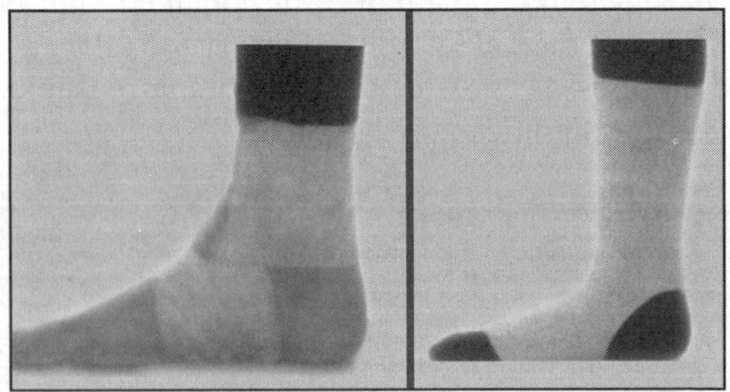

Fig. 1.38: Ankle strap

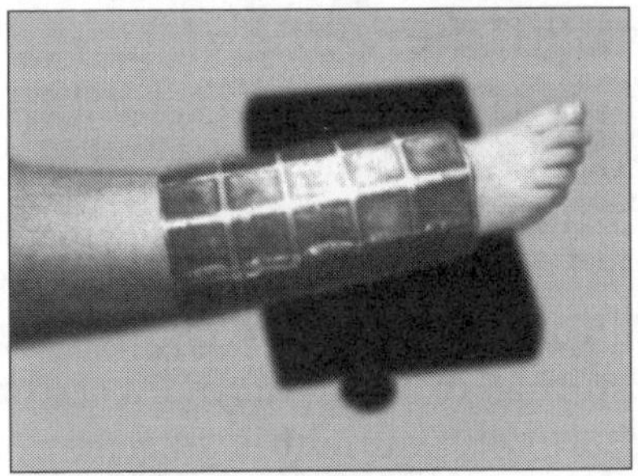

**Fig. 1.39:** The RICE regimen—rest, ice, compression and elevation

*Grade II sprain* : Long leg cast, range of motion exercises, strengthening exercises, etc. are helpful (Figs 1.40A and B).

*Grade III sprain* : Same lines as mentioned above and sometimes may rarely require surgical repair.

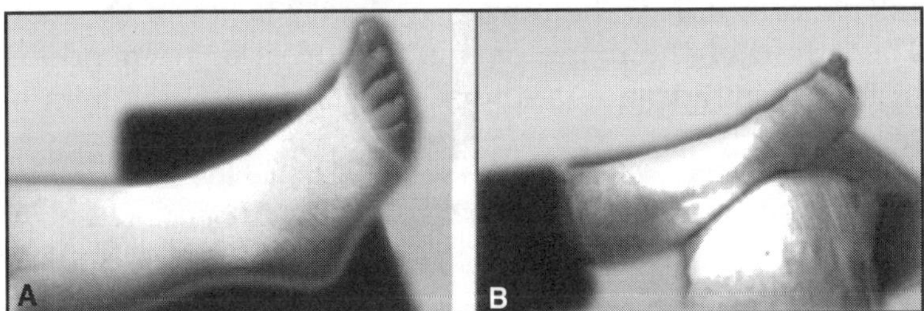

**Figs 1.40A and B:** (A) Compression bandaging, (B) elevation for ankle sprain

**Quick facts**

Treatment of acute ankle sprain in a nutshell (First 48 hours) (**PRICE** Regime) (*see* Fig. 1.12)

**P** – painkillers
**R** – rest
**I** – ice therapy
**C** – compression bandage (Jones bandage)
**E** – elevation at hip level.

## MEDIAL LIGAMENT SPRAIN

This is due to pronation eversion injury. In mild sprains, only the superficial part of the deltoid ligament is torn, but in severe forms, the deep part of the deltoid ligament is also torn resulting in a lateral talar tilt. If this exceeds more than 2 mm, significant alteration in the weight bearing mechanism takes place resulting in post-traumatic arthritis. For mild sprains, conservative treatment is sufficient and for severe sprains, surgical reduction and repair are considered.

**Do you know the sources of pain after acute ankle sprain?**

- Superficial peroneal nerve tension neuropathy.
- Anterior and lateral ankle impingement syndrome.
- Cuboid subluxation.

## TENDO-ACHILLES INJURY

There is no other stronger tendon in the body than the tendo-Achilles. Two powerful muscles, the gastrocnemius and the soleus form it. It is the powerful plantar flexor of the foot. The origin of the name of this tendon is of tremendous historical significance (*see* box).

**Do you know the interesting Greek story behind the Christening of this tendon as tendo-Achilles?**

Pleus and Thetis were the proud parents of the famous Greek hero, Achilles. His mother desired that his son should be so much fortified with strength that he remains indefatigable in the field of wars. Her coterie of well-wishers suggested to her that if she dips her son completely in the magical river Styx, no force on earth could ever defeat him. Completely obsessed with this thought, she immersed her son in that river by holding him with the tendon above the heel. Apparently, it seemed that she had achieved the impossible but was oblivious of the stark reality that the tendon area in the heel held by her remained undipped in the river and hence was deprived of the magical protection. A seemingly omnipotent Achilles met his Waterloo at the siege of Troy when he was slained by an injury to this tendon during the war. Ironically, though her mother could not make him immortal in war, she gave the idea to the orthopedic surgeons to name this tendon after his son and thus immortalized him.

*Note:* The moral of this story is whoever tries to play God will be vanquished!

## How is this strong tendon injured? Mechanism of Injury

### *Acute Rupture*

Any direct injury with a sharp object can injure this tendon. Interestingly, in our country, a curious mechanism of injury, thanks to the practice of Indian toilet system, is being described to the utter bewilderment and astonishment of the west. Let us take a closer look at this mechanism.

In the practice of the Indian toilet system, a person is prone to accidental slippage into the water closet of the toilet. Depending on the position of the foot, two types of injury may result:

- *High level injury (68%):* At the moment of slippage, if the foot is dorsiflexed, a high-level open injury is an inevitable outcome (about 3–4 cm above the insertion). However, the positive aspect is that these injuries will heal well after repair (Fig. 1.41A).
- *Low level injury (32%):* Here a panic-stricken patient tries to extricate his foot trapped in the closet in a plantar flexed position. This indiscretion leads to slicing of the tendon at a low level by the overhanging sharp edge of the closet. However, the problems are compounded due to poor healing after repair and due to sloughing of the skin (Fig. 1.41B).

### *Chronic Rupture*

This is due to gradual weakening of the tendon over the years. Spontaneous rupture may occur in such situations (*see* box).

## Clinical Features

In acute tears, the patient complains of pain and swelling in the region of the tendon. The patient is unable to walk.

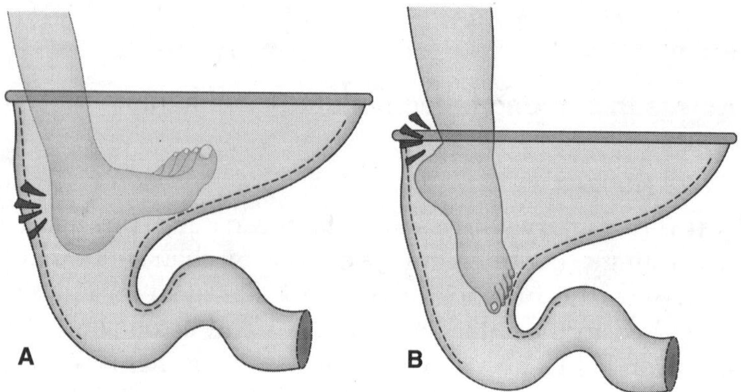


**Figs 1.41A and B:** Mechanism of injury of tendo-Achilles rupture: (A) High level injury, (B) low level injury

**Vital facts**

Predisposing factors leading to chronic TA rupture:

- Age more than 40 years, people involved in active athletics and sports
- Weakened athletes
- Previous history of tendonitis
- Loss of flexibility of tendo-Achilles.

However, in incomplete tears, when the patient is instructed to stand over the tiptoes, there will be a definite heel lag.

*Signs*

Tenderness can be elicited and a gap is felt during a complete tear. Dorsiflexon is exaggerated, but plantar flexion is diminished; but never totally absent due to the residual action of tibialis posterior, toe flexors and the peroneals.

## Clinical Tests

- Thompson's test is still the gold standard.
- O'Brien's needle test is also reliable.
- Tip toe test.

## X-ray of the Heel

- Lateral view of the heel will show soft tissue swelling around the heel.
- MRI scan helps to identify the tears more clearly (Fig. 1.42).

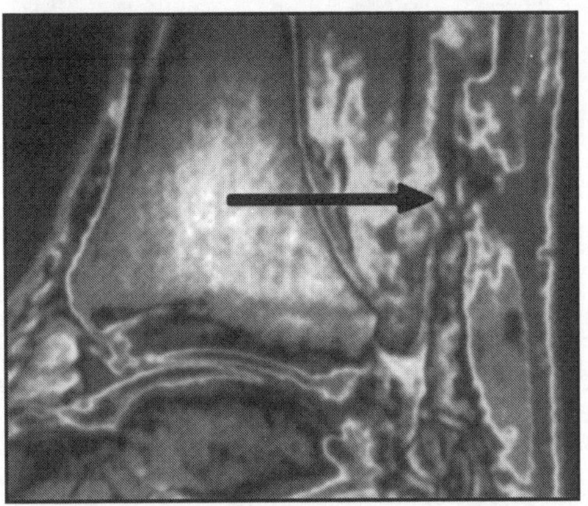

**Fig. 1.42:** MRI of tendo-Achilles rupture

**Interesting facts**

Do you know the common sites of rupture in chronic tears? It is 2–10 cm proximal to the insertion of the tendon in the OS Calcis: This area is weaker than other areas due to relative avascularity.

## Treatment

### *Conservative*

Immobilizing the ankle in slight plantar flexion for 6–8 weeks. Though the incidence of infection is less, recurrent ruptures are quite common. Hence, it is second best to surgery.

### *Surgery*

Direct surgical repair (Denholm's repair) and immobilization in a below knee plaster cast with slight plantar flexion is a better alternative. Though recurrent ruptures are less, the

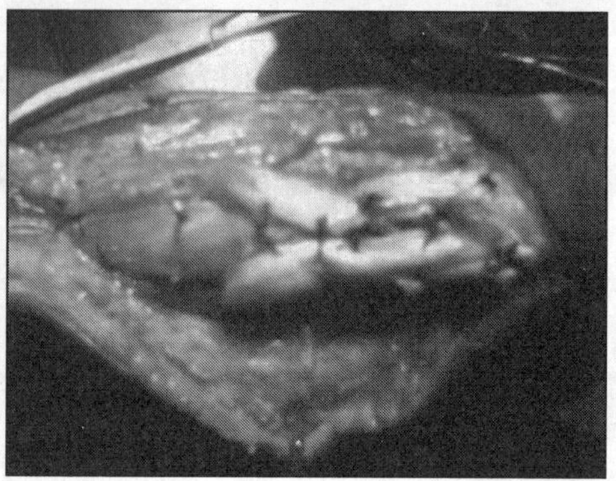

**Fig. 1.43:** Tendo-Achilles repair by Denholms method

chances of infections are high. Hence, extreme caution needs to be exercised to prevent the dreadful infection (Fig. 1.43).

## INJURIES OF THE FOOT

### INTRODUCTION

Injuries of the foot is quite common in athletes and other sports. It may range from minor sprain to major fractures of the foot bones. Let us now try to know some of the important foot injuries in sports.

### INJURIES OF THE FOREFOOT: PHALANGEAL FRACTURES

#### Salient Features

- This is the most common injury of the foot.
- Proximal phalanx is more commonly injured than all other phalanx.
- Proximal phalanx of the fifth toe is most commonly injured.

#### Mechanism of Injury

- Direct blow due to fall of a heavy object on the toes. This causes transverse or comminuted fractures.

- Indirect forces due to axial loading with secondary varus or valgus forces (stubbing injury). This leads to spiral or oblique fractures.

## Clinical Features

The patient presents with pain, swelling, limp and difficulty to wear the footwear.

## Investigation

Standard AP and lateral films of the forefoot help to make the diagnosis (Fig. 1.44).

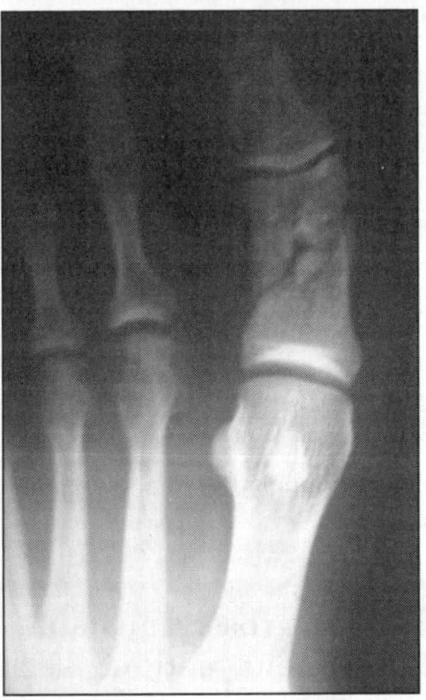

**Fig. 1.44:** Radiograph showing proximal phalanx fracture

## Classification (OTA)

*Group A:* Extra-articular and simple diaphyseal fractures.

*Group B:* Partial articular and diaphyseal wedge fractures.

*Group C:* Complex articular and diaphyseal shaft fractures. Each group is further subdivided into the position and pattern of fractures.

## Treatment

### *Nonoperative Treatment*

- *Immobilization only:* This is indicated for stable closed injuries with no intra-articular extension. The treatment consists of buddy taping and weight bearing with stiff shoes (Fig. 1.45).
- *Closed reduction:* This is indicated for displaced extra-articular or intra-articular fractures. The treatment consists of closed reduction and buddy taping to the medial toe.

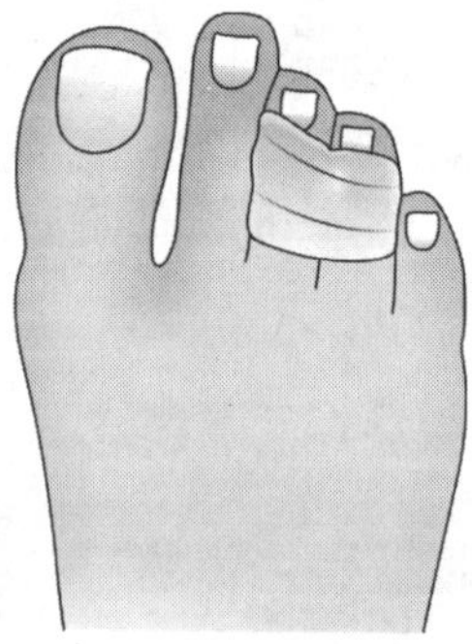

**Fig. 1.45:** Buddy taping for undisplaced phalangeal fractures of the toes

### *Operative Treatment*

This is indicated for grossly unstable intra-articular fractures. The treatment method of choice is closed reduction and percutaneous K-wire fixation or open reduction, K-wire or screw fixation.

## INTERPHALANGEAL JOINT DISLOCATIONS (IJD)

## Salient Features

- It is due to axial loading at the end of the digits.

- Majority occur in the proximal joint.
- Dorsal dislocation is more common.
- May be confused with phalangeal fractures.

### Clinical Features

Pain and swelling, stiffness of the toes, dorsoplantar thickening of the toe on palpation are the usual presentation.

### Investigation

*Plain X-rays:* AP and lateral views help to make the diagnosis.

### Treatment

Closed reduction with longitudinal traction along the toes with plantar flexion of the toes under digital block is the treatment method of choice. This is followed by buddy taping to the adjacent toe.

## METATARSOPHALANGEAL JOINT INJURIES

### First MTP Joint

#### *Salient Features*

- Most commonly injured.
- Most commonly affected during sports injury.
- Injuries vary from minor sprain to frank dislocations.

### Mechanism of Injury

Axial loading during:

- Hyperdorsiflexion (Turf toe)
- Hyperplantarflexion (Sand toe)
- Valgus and varus stress.

### Clinical Features

Pain over the great toe with weight bearing, tenderness over the MTP joint, ecchymosis, and test for both active and passive stability.

### Investigation

Weight bearing, AP and lateral views on plain X-rays.

### Classification

Type I : Dislocation with intact plantar plate.

Type II : Dislocation with partial disruption of plantar plate.

Type III : Dislocation with complete disruption of plantar plate.

Sprains are classified into Grades I, II and III, depending on the degree of tear.

### Treatment

*Nonoperative treatment:* For stable injuries, RICE regime.

*Operative treatment:* This is indicated for intra-articular fractures and significant avulsion fractures causing instability. These injuries need open reduction, internal fixation with ligament repair.

## INJURIES TO THE OTHER MTP JOINTS

These are hyperdorsiflexion and hyperplantarflexion injuries with axial loading and are rare. The treatment is essentially conservative for minor sprains. Dislocations are treated by closed reduction by finger traps to the affected toe for overcoming the gravitational force. This is successful in 50 percent of the cases. If this fails, open reduction and pinning may be required.

## SESAMOID BONE INJURIES

Two sesamoid bones are present within the flexor hallucis longus and flexor hallucis superficialis tendons of the great toe.

### Functions of Sesamoid Bones

- Shock absorber.
- Supports weight bearing function of the great toe.
- Protects the FHL tendon.

*Note:* Bipartite sesamoid bones are seen in 9–30 percent. Medial sesamoid is more commonly injured.

### Mechanism of Injury

- Due to the impact of the foot on a hard surface while the toes are dorsiflexed.
- Stress fracture due to repeated trauma (as in dancers; runners, etc.).

### Clinical Features

Pain, tenderness beneath the plantar surface of the sesamoid bone (Fig. 1.46), limp is present.

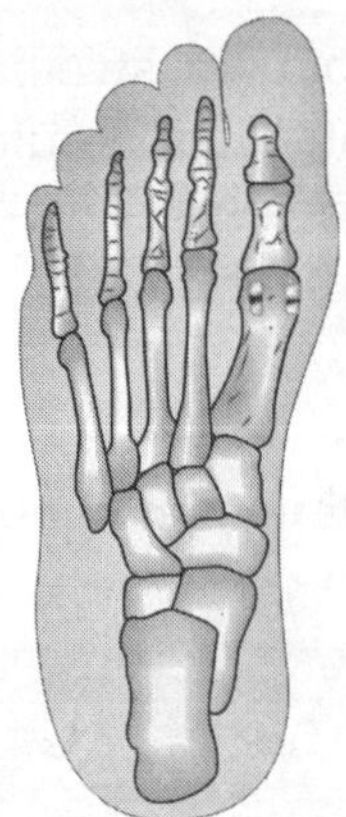

**Fig. 1.46:** Sesamoid bone fractures

### Investigations

- Plain X-ray–AP, lateral and tangential (sesamoid) views.
- CT scan or MRI is more accurate but expensive.

### Treatment

*Acute fractures:* Soft padding, strapping the MTP joint in neutral or in slightly plantar flexed position.

*Sesamoidectomy:* This is done if casting fails or if there is persisting pain.

## METATARSAL FRACTURES

### Mechanism of Injury

- Direct force—common, due to fall of a heavy object.
- Indirect force—Due to twisting forces, avulsion and spiral fractures are caused.
- Avulsion fractures are common at the base of the fifth metatarsal.
- Stress fractures are common at the II and III metatarsals (March fracture).

### Clinical Features

The patient complains of pain, swelling and tenderness over the dorsum of the foot. There could be considerable soft tissue swelling. Limp is present and pain in the foot increases with weight bearing.

### Radiograph

Plain X-ray with AP, lateral and oblique views help to make the diagnosis (Fig. 1.47).

### Classification (OTA)

Group A : Extra-articular and simple diaphyseal fractures.

Group B : Partial articular and diaphyseal wedge fractures.

Group C : Complex articular and diaphyseal shaft fractures.

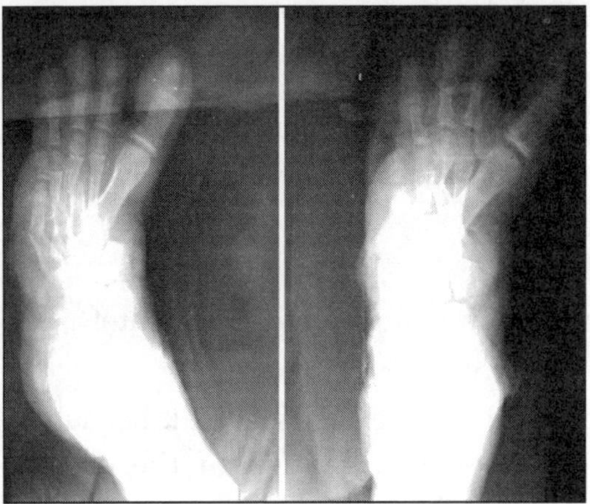

**Fig. 1.47:** Radiograph showing multiple metatarsal fractures

## Treatment

- *First metatarsal:*
  - *Nonoperative methods:* NWB below-knee plaster cast for 6–8 weeks for stable fractures with no loss of bone length.
  - *Operative methods:* Displaced and unstable fractures should be treated by closed reduction and percutaneous fixation with K-wires, screws only or with plate and screws.
- *Central metatarsals (2–4):* These injuries are more common than the first metatarsal.
  - *Nonoperative methods:* Fractures with < 10 mm long axis angulation and < 4 mm transition of shaft with hard or stiff-soled shoes for fractures with > 10 degree angulation and > 4 mm translation can be treated with closed reduction and gravity, traction or immobilization with hand or stiff-soled shoes.
  - *Operative methods:* Closed reduction and percutaneous K-wire fixation is done for unstable injuries and for multiple fractures.

## FIFTH METATARSAL INJURIES

### Mechanism of Injury

- *Direct force:* Rare and is seen in RTAs, sports, etc.
- *Indirect force:* Twisting force injury is more common.

### Classification

Fifth metatarsal fractures are divided into:

- Distal spiral or dancer's fracture.
- Proximal base fractures. These are further subdivided into:
  - *Pseudo-Jones fracture:* Tip of the styloid process (avulsion fracture).
  - *Jones fracture:* Metaphyseal fracture due to sudden adduction of the forefoot.
- Stress fracture of the proximal fifth metatarsal.

### Treatment

Nonoperative treatment is indicated for undisplaced and stable injuries and it consists of:

- Tip of the styloid process or Zone Injury—wearing hard sole or stiff shoes.
- Metaphyseal fractures (Jones)—below knee weight bearing plaster cast for 6–8 weeks.
- Diaphyseal fractures—NWB cast for 3 months.

## JONES FRACTURE

It is a fracture of the diaphysis of the fifth metatarsal bone approximately 1.5 cm above the tip of the tuberosity (Fig. 1.48A) at the metaphyseal junction.

### Mechanism of Injury

It is an avulsion fracture due to the pull of the peroneus brevis muscle. It is frequently encountered in athletes.

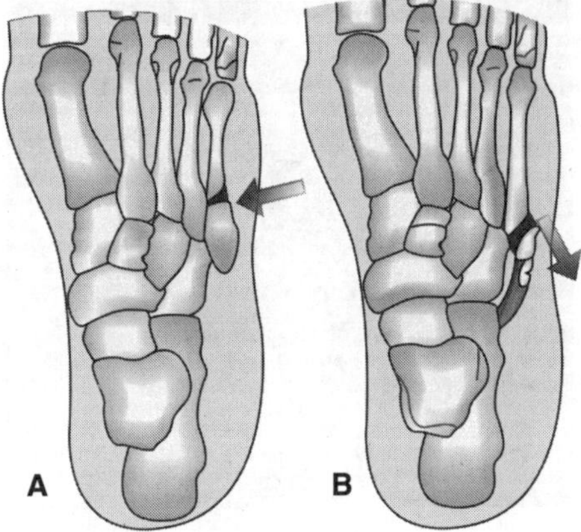


**Figs 1.48A and B:** (A) Jones fracture, (B) Avulsion fracture of the styloid process of 5th metatarsal bone

## Clinical Features

The patient complains of pain, swelling and limp. On examination, tenderness can be elicited over the base of the fifth metatarsal bone.

**Disturbing facts about Jones fracture**

- It is often confused with pseudo-Jones fracture.
- Delayed union and nonunion is a frequent occurrence due to the poor blood supply.
- Surgery may be required if there is nonunion.

**Do you know about pseudo-Jones fracture?**

- This is an avulsion fracture of the styloid process of the fifth metatarsal bone due to the pull of the peroneus brevis muscle (Fig. 1.48B).
- It heals readily and surgery is rarely required.

## Radiology

Radiograph of the foot helps to confirm the diagnosis. It shows a fuzzy periosteal reaction in the metadiaphyseal region after 7–10 days (Fig. 1.48C).

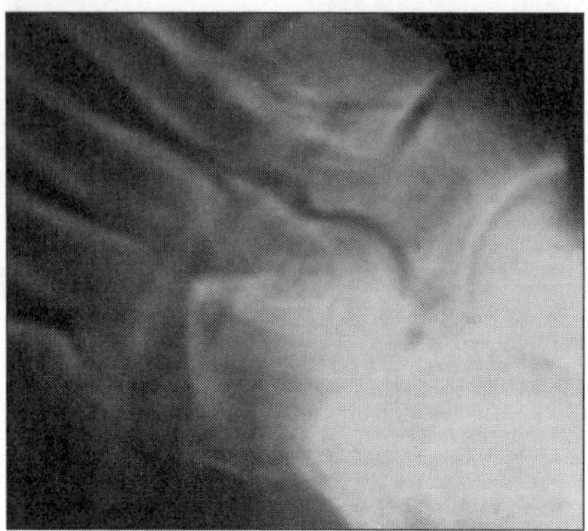

**Fig. 1.48C:** Jones fracture

### Treatment

Treatment is essentially conservative and consists of application of a below knee plaster cast for a period of 3–4 weeks.

## MARCH FRACTURE (INSUFFICIENCY FRACTURE)

This is a stress or fatigue fractures of the metatarsals particularly the II metatarsal bone (Fig. 1.49). It is more often encountered in military personnel who indulge in

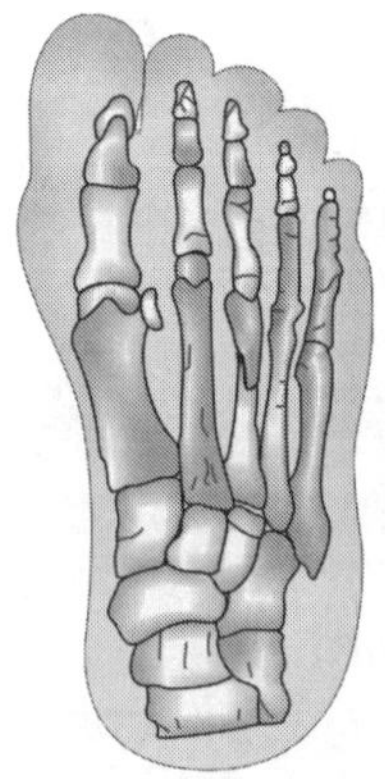

**Fig. 1.49:** March fracture

frequent and prolonged marching and hence its name. It is also seen in police officers, dancers, nurses, and surgeons, who require standing or dancing for a long duration. Radiograph helps in the diagnosis and the treatment is rest, NSAIDs, splints, elastic crepe bandage application, etc.

This is an important cause of chronic midfoot pain and it requires prompt identification and treatment.

## MIDFOOT INJURIES

Midfoot consists of the navicular, three cuneiform and cuboid bones with their intervening joints. This region of the foot is susceptible to injuries. Midfoot fractures are depicted in Flow chart 1.2.

### Mechanism of Injury

There are three common causes of midfoot fractures:

- *Twisting of the forefoot:* This usually occurs in an RTA due to forced foot abduction (twisting injury).
- *Axial loading of a fixed foot:* This can happen in two ways:
  - Fall on an extremely dorsiflexed foot (here an axial compression is applied to the heel).
  - Fall on an extremely ankle equinus (here axial compression is from the body weight).
- *Direct* crushing injuries as in industrial accidents.

### Treatment Goals

#### *Orthopedic Goal*

- To restore the keystone of the midfoot (i.e. the first and second metatarsal articulation with the medial cuneiform) as it provides stability between the midfoot and forefoot during gait.
- To maintain the medial longitudinal arch of the foot by restoring the length and alignment of the cuneiforms, cuboid and navicular bones. The longitudinal and transverse arches should be maintained as they control

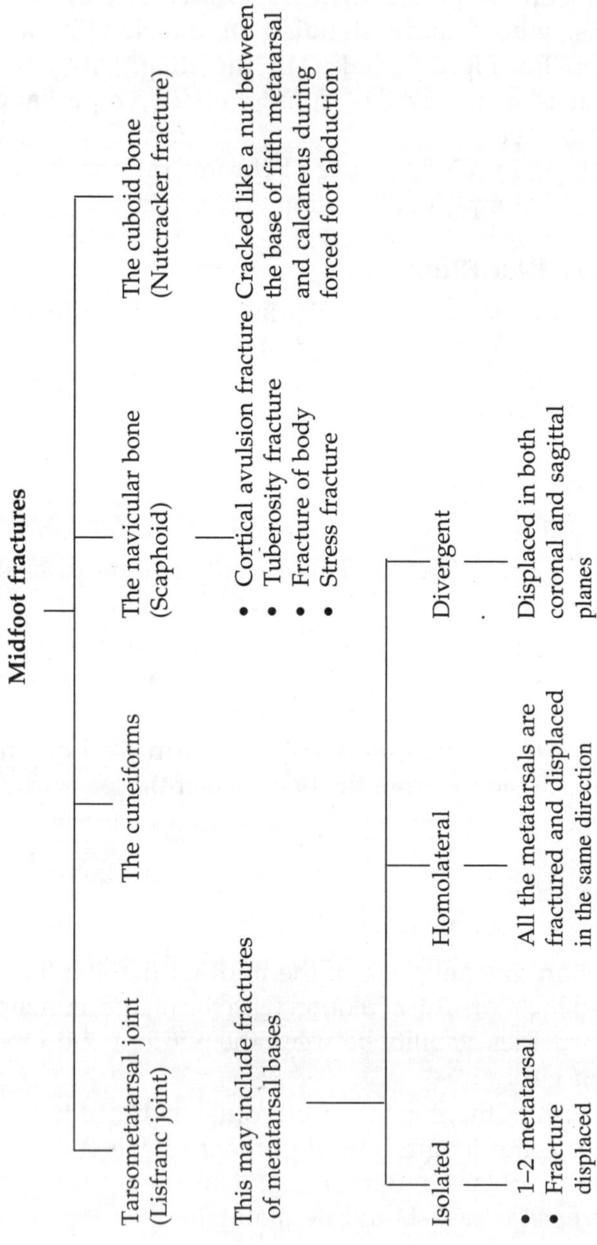


**Flow chart 1.2:** Midfoot fractures

the direct distribution of weight of the body or the foot during gait.
- To restore the Lisfranc joint complex.

*Note:* Midfoot extends between the Chopart's joint proximally to Lisfranc joint distally.

## NAVICULAR BONE FRACTURES

This is the keystone of the medial longitudinal arch of the foot (Fig. 1.50).

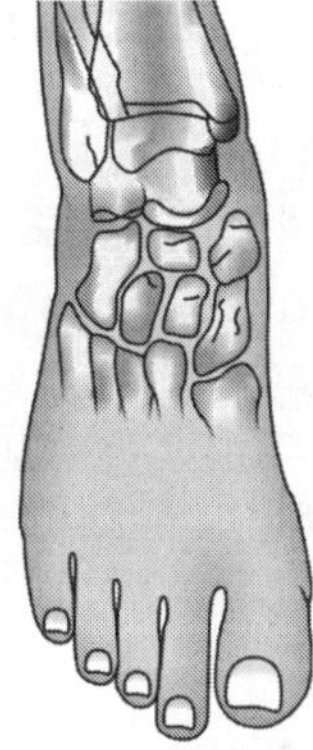

**Fig. 1.50:** Navicular bone fracture

### Mechanism of Injury

- *Direct blow:* Rare, can cause avulsion or crush injuries.
- *Indirect forces:* Due to fall from height, sports-related injuries or due to RTA.

### OTA Classification

*Group A:* Extra-articular fracture.
*Group B:* Involvement of the talonavicular joint.
*Group C:* Involvement of both talonavicular and talocuneiform joints.

Each group is further subclassified depending upon fracture types and position.

### Clinical Features

The patient complains of pain, swelling, and limp. Tenderness can be elicited over the navicular bone.

### Investigations

AP and lateral X-rays of the joint and CT scan give more reliable information about the fracture pattern.

### Treatment

- *Nonoperative treatment:* This is indicated in undisplaced fractures and in fracture with less than 2 mm displacement of the talonavicular joint. The treatment consists of short leg NWB cast for 6–8 weeks.
- *Operative treatment:* This is reserved for displaced fractures with > 2 mm separation. Fixation can be achieved most of the times by screw fixation alone. If more than 40 percent of the articular surface is damaged, talonavicular fusion should be considered.

### Complications

- Nonunion
- Avascular necrosis
- Collapse of the arch
- Post-traumatic osteoarthritis.

## CUBOID FRACTURES

### Mechanism of Injury

- Direct blow
- Indirect force: Forced plantar flexion and abduction (nutcracker effect).

### Clinical Features

The patient complains of dorsolateral pain, swelling and skin discoloration (Fig. 1.51).

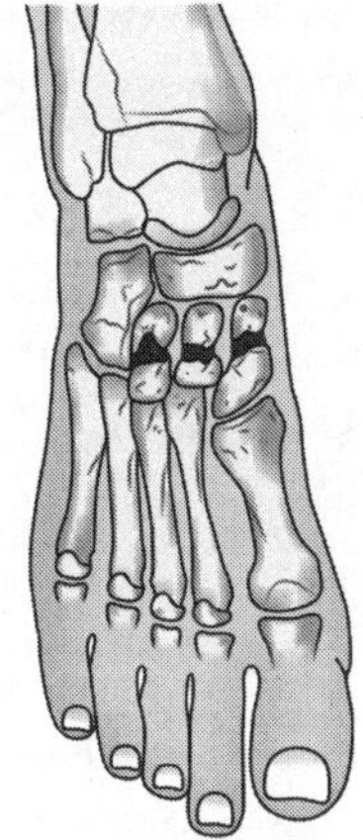

**Fig. 1.51:** Cuboid bone fracture

### Investigations

Plain X-ray with a medial oblique view and CT scan are the recommended investigations.

### Classification (OTA) (For medical readers)

*Group A* : Extra-articular.

*Group B* : Partly intra-articular involving either the calcaneocuboid or the metatarsocuboid joints.

*Group C* : Completely intra-articular involves both the joints.

Each group is further classified depending upon the fracture pattern and position.

### Treatment

*Nonoperative method:* This is indicated in undisplaced and in fractures < 2 mm separation. The treatment of choice is a below knee cast for 6–8 weeks.

*Operative method:* For displaced fractures, open reduction and K-wire fixation is indicated. External fixation is recommended for the nutcracker fracture.

*Note:* Cuboid syndrome is a painful subluxation of the calcaneocuboid joint.

## CUNEIFORM INJURIES

These are rare injuries and are usually due to indirect forces. More commonly, they are associated with injuries to the tarsometatarsal joints (Fig. 1.52).

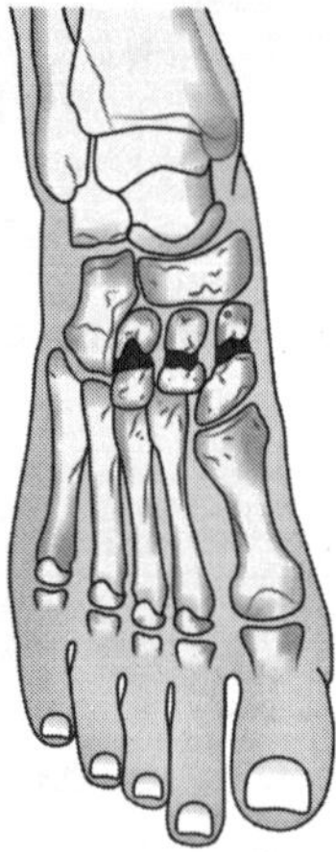

**Fig. 1.52:** Cuneiform bone fractures

### Clinical Features

Pain, swelling, tenderness, limp and pain on weight bearing.

### Investigations

Plain X-ray (AP, lateral, oblique views) with CT scan of the foot.

### Classification (OTA) (For medical readers)

*Group A* : Extra-articular.
*Group B* : Partly intra-articular (involves other navicular cuneiform or metatarsal cuneiform joints).
*Group C* : Involves both articular surfaces.

### Treatment

*Nonoperative:* Short leg cast for 6 to 8 weeks for undisplaced fractures.

*Operative:* For displaced fractures, open reduction and internal fixation with pins or screws.

## TARSOMETATARSAL INJURIES (These are called Lisfranc injuries)

Lisfranc joint consists of three cuneiform metacarpal articulations and two cuboid metatarsal articulations of the fourth and fifth metatarsals. It represents the transition bone between the midfoot and the forefoot.

### Mechanism of Injury

- *Direct injury:* This is rare and is due to crush injury or direct blow on the dorsum of the foot.
- *Indirect injury:* This is more common and three varieties are described (Figs 1.53A and B):
  - Axial loading to the foot in fixed equinus (e.g. football injuries).
  - Axial loading in descending stairs.
  - Axial loading following fall from height.

The associated injuries could be fracture of second metatarsal (most common), fractures of cuneiforms, cuboids, metatarsals and lateral ligament injuries.

### Clinical Features

- Pain in the tarsometatarsal area.
- Passive dorsiflexion or plantar flexion produces pain.
- Single limb heel lift produces pain in the midfoot.
- Plantar ecchymosis.

### Investigations

- Plain X-ray in weight bearing position (AP, lateral and 30° medial oblique position) (Fig. 1.54).

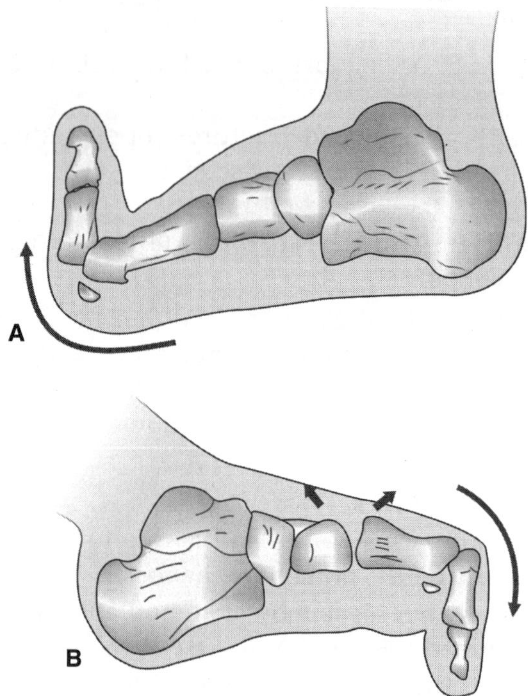


**Figs 1.53A and B:** Mechanisms of Lisfranc injury

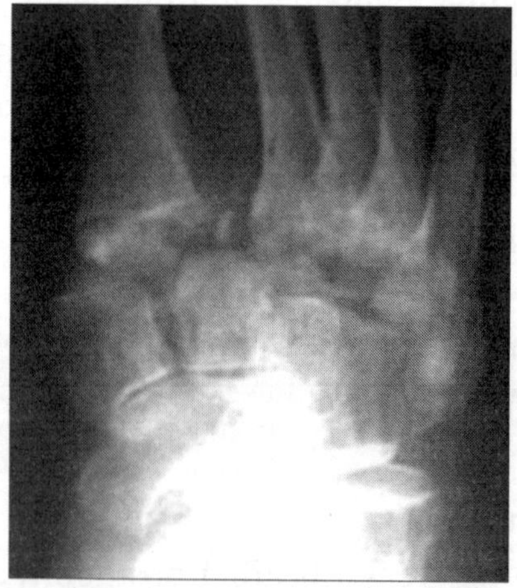

**Fig. 1.54:** Lisfranc fracture

- CT scan provides better visualization and is more accurate in analyzing the injuries.

**CLASSIFICATION (OTA)** (Figs 1.55A to C)
(For Medical Readers)

- *Type I:* Anterior dislocation 1st ray, dorsal and plantar dislocations of the lesser rays.

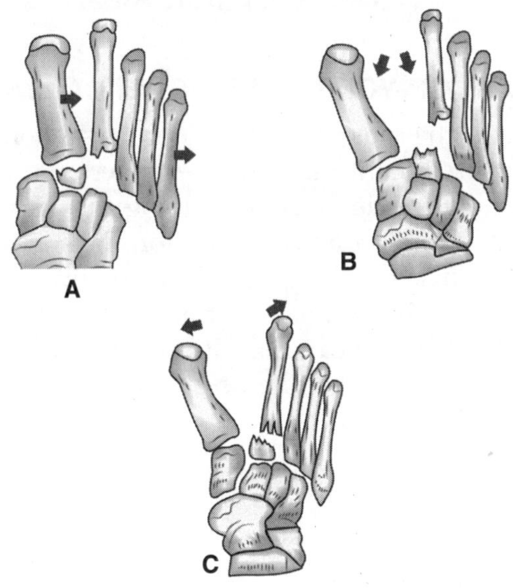


**Figs 1.55A to C:** Different types of Lisfranc injury (A) Type I, (B) Type II, (C) Type III

- *Type II:* Divergent dislocation.
- *Type III:* Homolateral dislocation (medial or lateral).

### Treatment

*Nonoperative methods:* This is indicated for sprains and for < 2 mm displacement of tarsometatarsal joint in any plane. The treatment of choice is a below knee POP cast for 6–8 weeks. For sprains—RICE regime.

*Operative methods:* For displaced injuries, closed reduction and internal fixation. With K-wires or screws is indicated for displacement < 50 percent. For more than 50 percent displacement, primary fusion is indicated. Open reduction or internal fixation is indicated for widely displaced fractures (Fig. 1.14).

## HINDFOOT INJURIES

### FRACTURE OF YOUR HEEL BONE, CALCANEUM

Calcaneus is the most often fractured tarsal bone. No ideal method of treatment has been described yet. It is a 'soft' bone residing inside your heel doing the 'hard' jobs like weight transmission and locomotion. It is a 'small' bone cut out for 'big' challenging and difficult roles. Because of its location it is infrequently fractured (except in a select few, see box) but because of its function it is a seat for many a problem in life like heel pain, calcaneal spur, etc. (*see* Regional disorders).

**Interesting Facts**

The unlucky few, who are more prone for calcaneal fractures are the ones who are more likely to fall from height and land on the feet like:

- Construction workers of high rise buildings.
- Electrical and telephone linemen working atop the poles.
- Casual laborers engaged in plucking the tender coconuts from the lanky coconut trees,
- Athletes involved in high jump and long jumps etc.
  Last but not the least, thieves who jump down the houses, after burglary to escape being caught by the police or the public!

#### Functions

- Supports weight of the body.
- Acts as a springboard for locomotion.

### Structure

It has a thin cortical shell except at the posterior tuberosity. Two types of trabecular pattern are described.

- *Traction trabeculae:* This radiates from the inferior cortex.
- *Compression trabeculae:* Converge to support anterior and posterior facets.

### Vital Angles

In the lateral view of the radiograph, two angles are important:

*Böhler's angle:* This is the angle between lines drawn from anterior articular process to the posterior tuberosity. The tuber angle is 25–40° (Fig. 1.56).

*Crucial angle of "Gissane":* The lateral process of talus is wedged in this angle (Fig. 1.57).

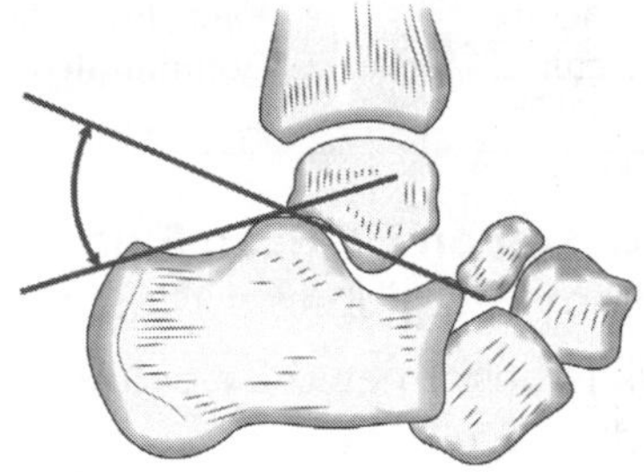

**Fig. 1.56:** Tuber joint angle (Böhler's angle)

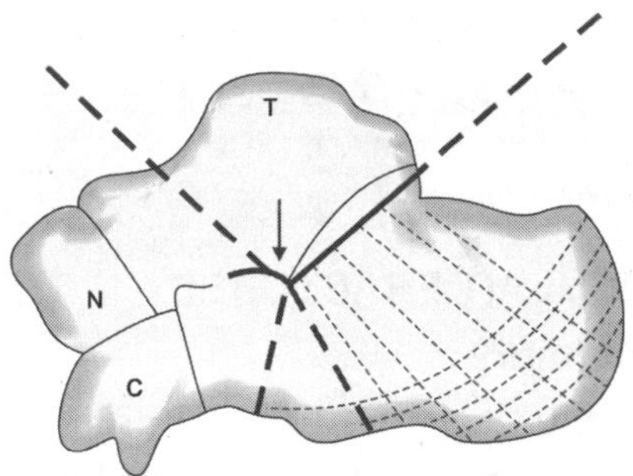


**Fig. 1.57:** Gissane angle

Axial compressive forces with talus acting as a bursting wedge will disrupt the subtalar joint.

Restoration of the above two angles is the aim of the treatment.

## CLASSIFICATION (For medical readers only)

### Essex-Lopresti's Classification

This is the most accepted classification for fracture calcaneum. It consists of extra-articular fractures (less common accounting for only 25% of the cases) and intra-articular fractures, which is more common (Fig. 1.58A and Table 1.7).

**Table 1.7:** Types of calcaneal fractures

| *Extra-articular (25-30%)* | *Intra-articular (70-75%)* |
|---|---|
| • Fracture anterior process | • Undisplaced fracture |
| • Fracture tuberosity | • Tongue-shaped fractures |
| • Medial process fracture | • Joint depression |
| • Fracture sustentaculum talus and body | • Comminuted fracture |

### Classification Based on CT Scan Findings (Intra-articular) (Crossby-Fitzgibban's Classification)

*Type I* : This is best treated by below-knee plaster cast

Type I : Undisplaced fracture.

Type II : Displaced intra-articular fractures of the posterior facet (< 2 mm).

Type III : Comminuted fractures.

*Note:*
Type I : Nonoperative treatment.
Type II: Operative treatment.

## EXTRA-ARTICULAR FRACTURES

### Mechanism of Injury

*Twisting forces* cause many of the extra-articular fractures. *Fall from height* with landing on the heels causes vast majority of intra-articular fractures (Fig. 1.58A).

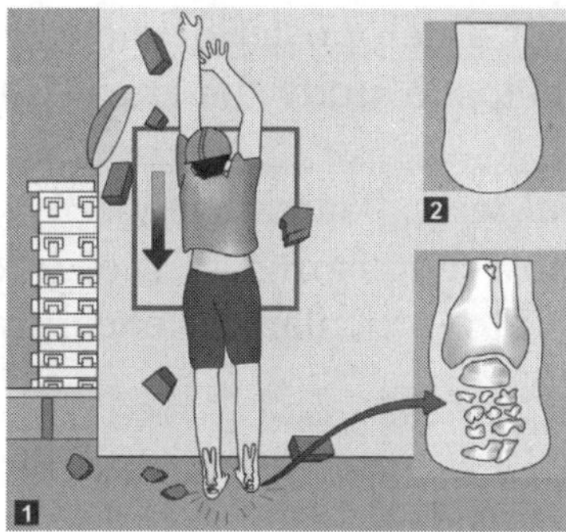

**Fig. 1.58A:** (1) Fall from height causes intra-articular fracture of calcaneum, (2) Broadening of the heel

**Vital facts**

- Bilateral fractures are seen in 5–9 percent of cases.
- Ten percent cases have compression fracture of dorsal or lumbar vertebral bodies.
- Twenty-six percent are associated with other injuries of the lower limbs.

**Clinical features:** Patient complains of

- Pain
- Swelling,
- Limp and
- Painful restricted movements of the subtalar and the midfoot joints.

## Radiography (Fig. 1.58B)

Plain X-rays of the foot with the following three views are recommended:

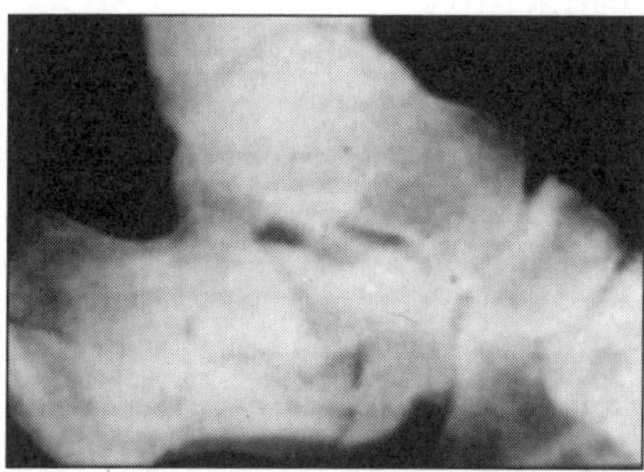

**Fig. 1.58B:** Radiograph showing calcaneum fracture

- Dorsoplantar or anteroposterior view (Fig. 1.59A).
- Lateral view helps to study the crucial angle of Gissane (Fig. 1.59B).
- Axial calcaneal view (Harris view).
- CT scan is now emerging as the gold standard in evaluation of intra-articular calceneal fractures.

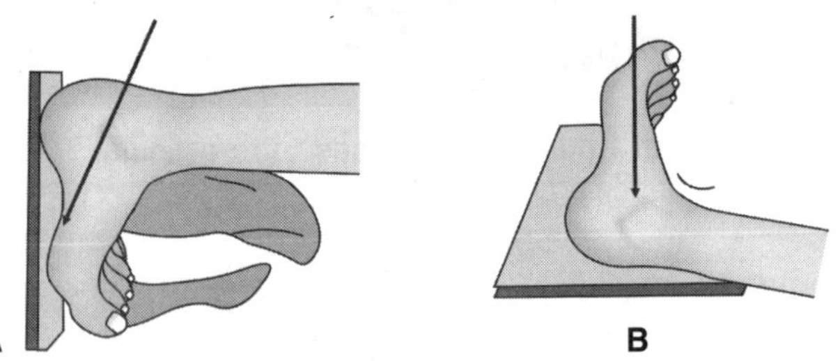


**Figs 1.59A and B:** Radiographic views: (A) Dorsoplantar view, and (B) Lateral view

### Classification of Extra-articular Fractures

- Anterior fracture of the anterior process.
- Middle:
  - Body fracture.
  - Fracture of sustentaculum tali.
  - Lateral calcaneal process fracture.
  - Peroneal tubercle fracture.
- Posterior:
  - Tuberosity fracture.
  - Medial calcaneal tubercle fracture.

### How to manage this fracture? Treatment

*Extra-articular Fractures*

- Fracture of anterior process:
  - Avulsion fracture—short leg cast (Fig. 1.60).
  - Compression fracture should be reduced and fixed with K-wire or screw.

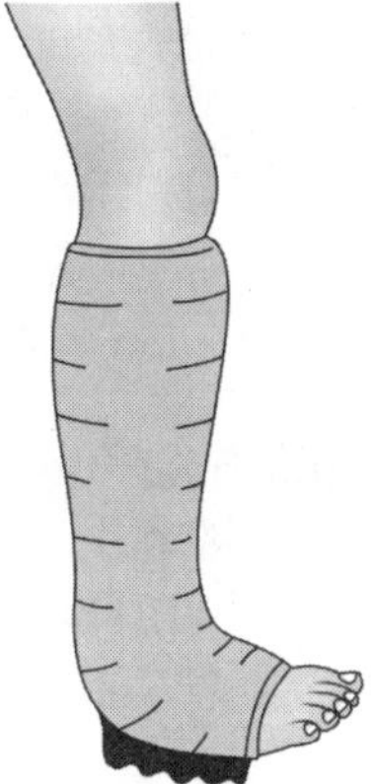

**Fig. 1.60:** Short leg POP cast with walking heel for calcaneal fracture

- Fracture tuberosity:
  - Undisplaced fracture—short leg cast.
  - Displaced fracture—open reduction and internal fixation.
- Fracture medial calcaneal process:
  - Undisplaced fracture—plaster cast.
  - Displaced—open reduction with medial lateral compression and internal fixation.
- Fracture sustentaculum tali:
  - Undisplaced—plaster cast.
  - Displaced—open reduction and casting.
- Fracture of the body not involving the subtalar joint: Responds well to conservative treatment.

## INTRA-ARTICULAR FRACTURES

These account for 60 percent of all tarsal injuries and 75 percent of all calcaneal fractures.

### Mechanism of Injury

*Fall from height:* Lateral process of talus acts as a wedge and is forced through the Gissane's angle resulting in four fracture patterns:

- Undisplaced.
- Tongue shaped.
- Joint depression.
- Comminuted.

## Clinical Features

- Pain and swelling of the heel, the patient is unable to bear weight, stand or walk, pain and difficulty during inversion and eversion of the heel.

## Clinical Signs

- Swelling over the heel.
- Tenderness over the heel.
- Lateral heel compression test elicits pain (Fig. 1.61).
- Broadening of the heel (Fig. 1.58A)
- Horseshoe swelling on either side the tendo-Achilles.
- Distance between the heel and malleoli is reduced.

## Radiography

Plain X-rays of the foot as in extra-articular fractures (Fig. 1.62).

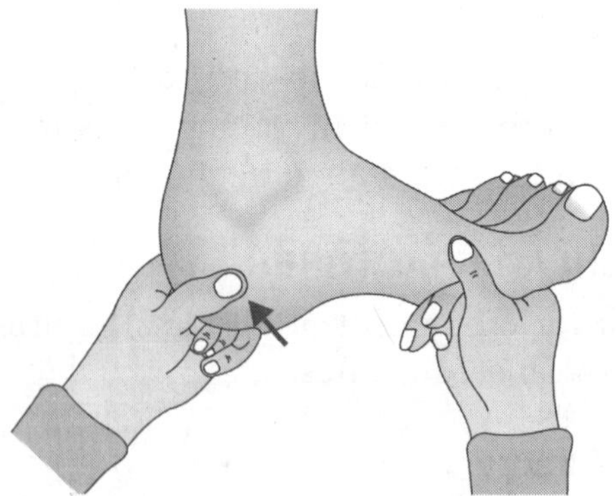

**Fig. 1.61:** Heel compression test for diagnosing undisplaced or stress fracture of calcaneum

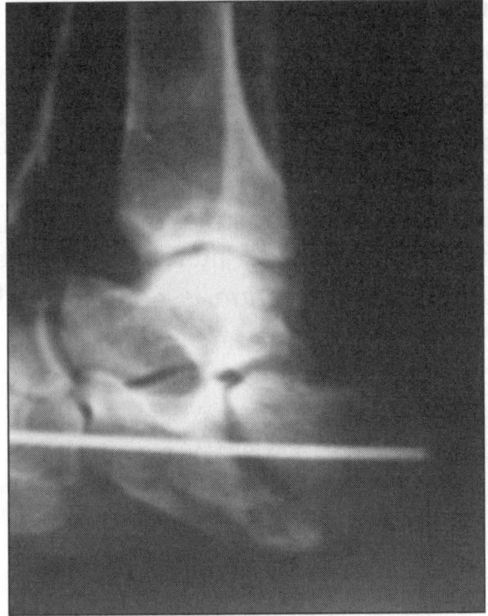

**Fig. 1.62:** Radiograph showing intra-articular calcaneum fracture

CT scan is now emerging as the gold standard in evaluation of intra-articular calceneal fractures.

## Treatment

### *Conservative*

The following are the basic methods of treatment:

- No reduction and early motion consists of:
  - Elastocrepe bandage application.
  - Foot elevation.
  - Weight bearing at the end of 12 weeks.
- Closed reduction and fixation.

*Goals*

- Restore congruity of the subtalar joint.
- Restore Böhler's angle.
- Restore normal width of the calcaneum.

## Omoto Technique of Calcaneal Fracture Reduction (Fig. 1.63)

*Common Steps of Reduction*

- Under anesthesia (general or spinal), the patient is prone and knee is flexed to 90°.
- With the assistant supporting the thigh, the surgeon compresses the medial and lateral sides of the heel.
- Strong longitudinal traction is now applied along the direction of the leg.
- Varus or valgus force is now applied depending on the displacement.
- Lastly the calceneal tuberosity is manipulated in position.
- Compression bandage is finally applied.

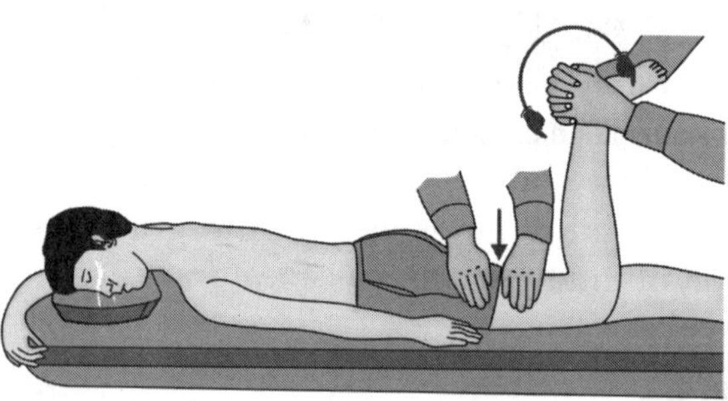

**Fig. 1.63:** Method of closed reduction of calcaneal fractures (Omoto technique)

**Essex-Lopresti method** of lifting the fragment with an axial percutaneous pin and retention with K-wires is done (Figs 1.64A and B).

## Surgery

Severely comminuted and depressed fracture with subchondral defects requires open reduction and internal fixation with cancellous bone graft to fill the gap. Recently, for this purpose, alternatively, biocompatible and less reabsorbable nanocrystalline calcium phosphate cement

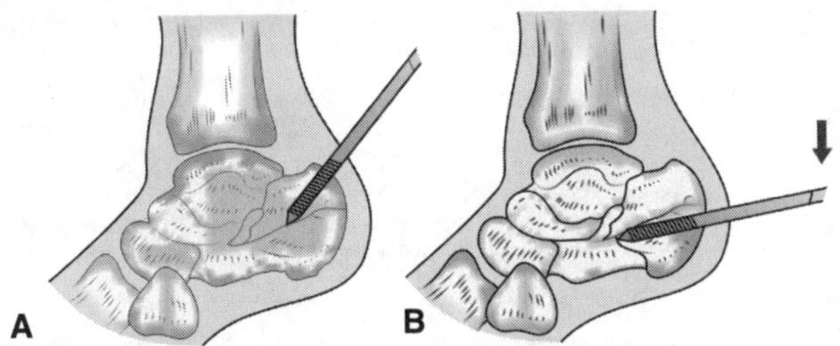


**Figs 1.64A and B:** Essex-Lopresti method of reduction of calcaneal fractures: (A) Disimpaction, (B) Elevation

called Bioban is being tried with successful results in some centers.

Open reduction and internal fixation with plate and screws are difficult and are rarely adopted.

## Complications

- Nonunion is rare due to the cancellous nature of the bone.
- Malunion is more common.
- *Heel pain:* The source of heel pain could be from:
  - Subtalar joint due to post-traumatic osteoarthritis.
  - Peroneal tendonitis due to stenosing tenovaginitis of the peroneal tendons.
  - Bone spurs due to malunion of fracture and disruption of fat pad of the heel.
  - Arthritis of calcaneocuboid joint is a major source of pain.
  - Nerve entrapment is rare. Medial or lateral plantar branches of posterior tibial nerve or sural nerve may be entrapped due to soft tissue scarring.

# 2

# Spinal Injuries in Sports

## INJURIES OF THE CERVICAL SPINE

Injuries of the cervical spine are dangerous; and if associated with neurological damage, the results can be devastating. Though diagnostic and treatment methods have vastly improved over years, still injuries of the cervical spine pose the greatest challenge to the skill and acumen of orthopedic and neurosurgeons.

Jefferson pointed out two areas commonly involved in cervical spine injuries, $C_{1-2}$ and $C_{5-7}$. According to Meyer, $C_2$ and $C_5$ are commonly involved. Neurological damage is seen in 40 percent of cases. In 10 percent of cases, radiographs are normal.

### Causes

*Fall from height:* It is the most common cause in developing countries.

*Diving injuries:* Diving into water with insufficient depth or in an inebriated condition.

*Road traffic accidents (RTAs):* Common cause in developed countries, e.g. whiplash injury (Fig. 2.1).

*Gunshot injuries*: These injure the cervical spine and the cord directly.

### Mechanism of Injury (Figs 2.2A to D)

*Pure flexion force:* For example, compression fracture of vertebral body, e.g. fall from height.

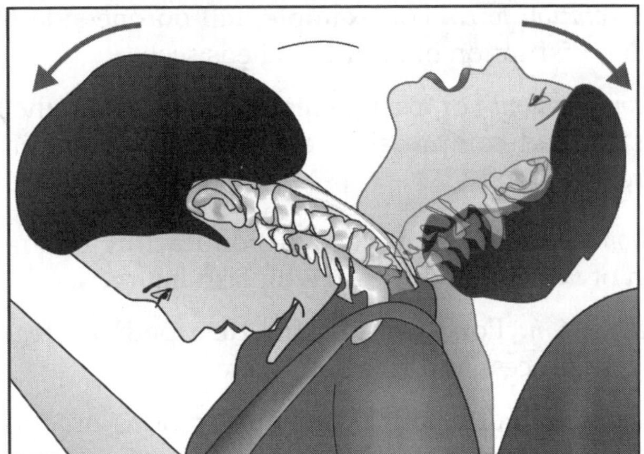

**Fig. 2.1:** Whiplash injury: Due to sudden deceleration, forceful hyperextension is followed by flexion of the neck

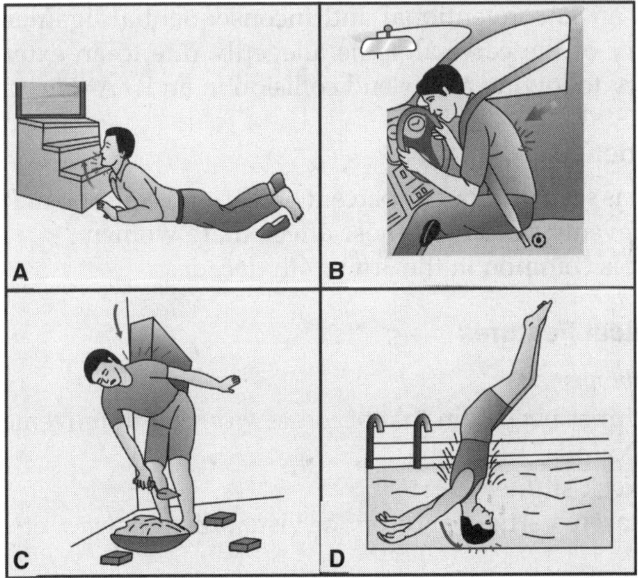

**Figs 2.2A to D:** Common mechanism of cervical spine injuries: (A) Hyperextension injury, (B) Flexion extension injury, (C) Flexion rotation injury, (D) Hyperflexion injury

*Flexion rotation force*: For example, fall on one side of the shoulder, disruption of facet capsule is seen.

*Axial compression:* For example, fall of an object on the head results in load compression, e.g. explosive comminuted fracture of C5 body.

*Extension force:* For example, avulsion fracture of superior margin of vertebral body, e.g. whiplash injury.

*Lateral flexion:* For example, fracture pedicle, fracture transverse process and facet joints, etc.

*Direct injuries*: For example, fracture spinous process and body. Due to assault, gunshot injury, etc.

## WHIPLASH INJURY (Syn: Acceleration injury, cervical sprain syndrome, soft tissue neck injury)

### Definition

It is an unconventional and inconsequential ligamentous injury of the cervical spine allegedly due to an extension injury following a rear-end collision in an RTA (Fig. 2.1).

### Incidence

- It is seen in about 25 percent of rear-end collision of RTAs.
- Seventy percent of those affected are women.
- It is common in the 3rd or 4th decades.

### Clinical Features

*Symptoms*

- Upper neck pain that becomes worse with movement.
- Occipital headache.
- Neck stiffness.
- Rarely vertigo, auditory or visual disturbances, etc.

*Signs*

- Decreased range of neck movements.
- Neck muscle spasm is seen.

*Note:* Symptoms appear within 48 hours of injury and 57 percent recover within three months. Final state is reached by one year.

### Investigations

X-rays are usually normal. MRI helps to make a diagnosis.

### Treatment

It is mainly conservative and consists of the following:

- *Drugs:* NSAIDs, muscle relaxants, etc. are given.
- *Collars:* These are recommended for the first three days.
- Short arc active movements are slowly begun.
- Active ROM exercises are slowly commenced.
- After the pain subsides, isometric strengthening exercises are slowly commenced.
- Other modalities take ultrasound, traction, manipulation, massage, etc. also helps.

### Allen's Classification of Cervical Spine Fractures (Figs 2.3A to D)

*Compressive flexion (5 stages):* Ranges from blunting of anterosuperior vertebral margin to posterior displacement

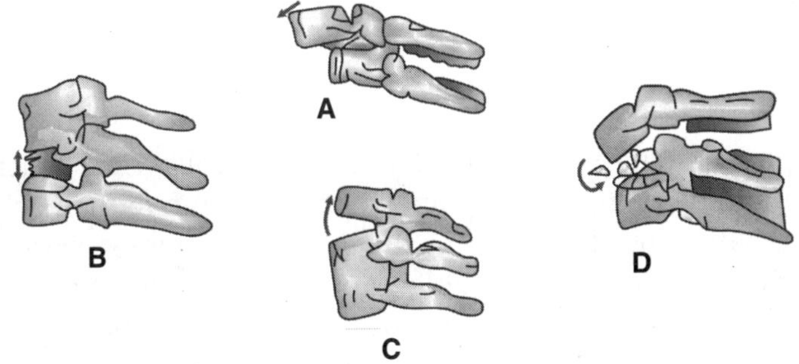


**Figs 2.3A to D:** Cervical spine injuries: (A) Distraction injury, (B) Compression injury, (C) Hyperextension injury, (D) Compression and distraction injury

into the spinal canal. It is usually a stable fracture but may become unstable if compression is more than 50 percent.

*Vertical compression (3 stages):* Ranges from fracture of superior or inferior endplate with centrum fracture of the vertebral body. Stable fracture if compression is less than 50 percent of the vertebral body.

*Distractive flexion (4 stages):* Ranges from failure of posterior ligamentous complex to full-width vertebral body displacement. This is an unstable fracture.

*Compression extension (5 stages):* Ranges from unilateral vertebral arch fracture to bilateral vertebral arch fracture with full-vertebral body displacement anteriorly. It is unstable.

*Distractive extension:* Ranges from failure of anterior ligament complex to posterior ligament complex. This is also an unstable fracture.

*Lateral flexion:* Ranges from asymmetric compression and ipsilateral vertebral arch to fracture without displacement and with displacement. May become unstable.

*Note:* All unstable cervical spine fractures have a high incidence of neurological damage.

## Clinical Features

The patient usually gives history of trauma following which there will be pain, swelling and inability to move the neck. There will be tenderness over the involved spinous process and there could be a palpable gap. There may be signs of neurological involvement. Determine the level of cord injury by examining the affected spine (*see* box). The injuries to the spinal cord at the cervical region can manifest in the following ways:

### *Concussion*

This is a state of spinal shock and there will be sensory loss, flaccid paralysis, visceral paralysis, reflexes are in abeyance and anal reflex is absent. By 8 hours, concussion is known to regress; and by 8–10 days, there is complete recovery.

### *Nerve Root Involvement*

Individual nerve roots could be affected at their respective intervertebral foramen. All the features of peripheral nerve injury with LMN type of lesion are seen. The myotome and the dermatome should be assessed to know the root involvement.

***Cord involvement*** could be:
*Complete:* This leads to quadriplegia or quadriparesis.
*Incomplete:* Here the central cord, lateral cord, anterior or posterior cord could be involved.

## Other Examinations

*Rectal sensation:* Loss of sensation around the anus.

*Rectal motor:* Sphincter contracts, over a gloved finger.

*Bulbocavernosus reflex:* Involves S1, S2 and S3 nerve roots. Squeeze the glans penis, anal sphincter contracts around the gloved finger.

Initially, following the injury, the above reflexes are absent, indicating spinal shock. Usually, it returns within 24 hours. If not a presumptive diagnosis and determination of a root or cord lesion is made. A diagnosis of a complete or incomplete syndrome is documented.

## Investigations

*Radiography:* Lateral view is important (Fig. 2.4). If an adequate lateral radiography reveals no fracture or dislocation, then a complete radiographic examination

**Cord concussion**

A state of "spinal shock", i.e. temporary electrical dysfunction.

**Features**

- Sensory loss.
- Flaccid paralysis.
- Visceral paralysis.
- Reflexes are in abeyance.
- Anal reflex lost (anal wink lost).

**Usually**

- Eight hours later concussion regresses.
- Seven to ten days later complete recovery. If the reflexes, do not return within 24 hours to 10 days a diagnosis of complete cord transection is made.

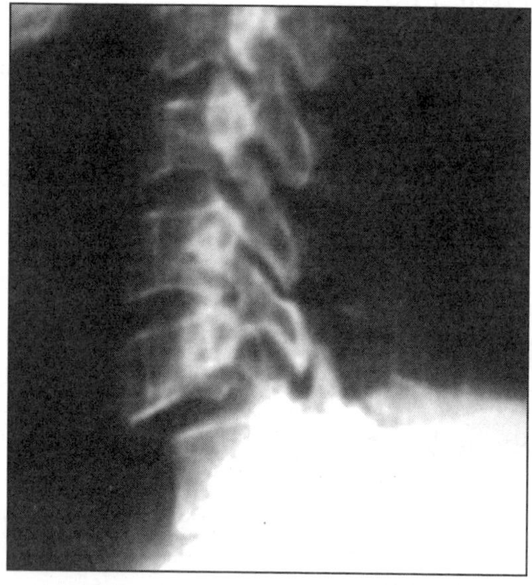

**Fig. 2.4:** Radiograph showing fracture dislocation of C6 over C7

including anteroposterior, open mouth and oblique projections are performed.

*Myelography* is of value in incomplete lesion who fails to show progressive improvement.

*CT scan* makes an accurate diagnosis of hidden fracture. It is not helpful in assessing the soft tissue injury.

*MRI evaluates* cord injuries better. MRI is found to be very reliable and helpful in assessing the bony, soft tissue damages and injury to the cord very accurately.

*General laboratory investigations*: Like Hb percentage, blood group, bleeding time, clotting time, electrolyte status, etc. are done.

**Treatment facts**

**Goals of treatment of cervical spine injury**

- Realign the spine.
- Prevent further neurological damage.
- Aid neurological recovery.
- Obtain and maintain spinal stability.
- Aim at early functional recovery.

## Treatment Methods

### *At the Accident Site*

Resuscitation and transport is important. In a person lying still without using his neck after an RTA, a cervical spine injury is always suspected until proved otherwise.

The patient is transported with utmost care over a stretcher to the hospital. All unnecessary neck movements should be totally avoided. If the patient needs resuscitation, it has to be carried out with a lot of care.

### *At the Hospital*

*Nonoperative treatment:* Most cases can be treated nonoperatively by halo vest, four postcervical collars, Minerva jacket, cervical collars, etc. (Figs 2.5A to C).

#### *Indications*

- Stable cervical spine with no neurological injury. A rigid cervical brace or halo for 8–12 week is usually sufficient.

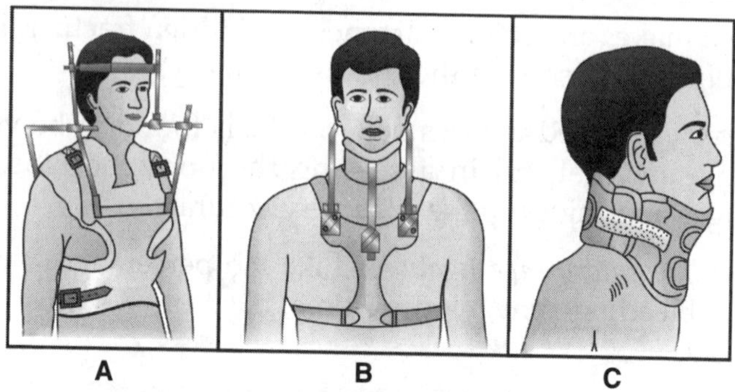


**Figs 2.5A to C:** Methods of cervical immobilization: (A) Halo-vest traction, (B) Four post cervical collar, (C) Cervical collar

- Stable compression fracture of vertebral bodies and undisplaced fracture of laminae, lateral masses or spinous process.
- Unilateral facet dislocations reduced in traction may be immobilized in a halo vest for 8–12 weeks.

***Skeletal traction:*** Reduction with traction is done for unstable fracture (Fig. 2.6). Urgency of reduction is based on neurological loss (Table 2.1). Traction is given for 3–6

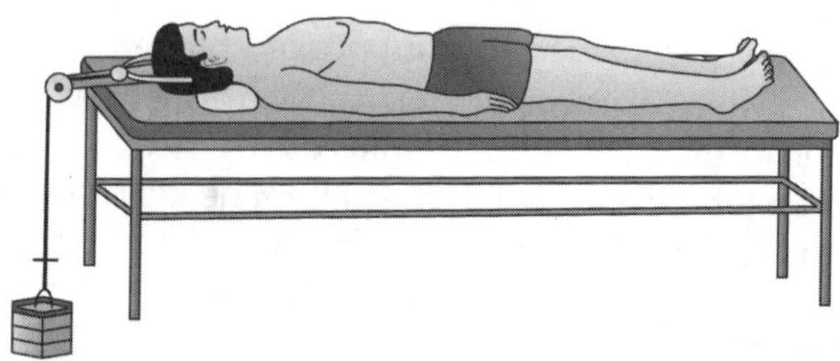

**Fig. 2.6:** Skeletal traction applied through Crutchfield tongs

weeks and once satisfactory reduction is achieved, the patient is mobilized with a collar, corset or jacket.

*Halo Vest Immobilization:* Many unstable cervical spine injuries can initially be managed by cervical traction through

**Table 2.1:** Skeletal traction

| Neurologic loss | No neurologic loss |
|---|---|
| ↓ | ↓ |
| Urgent skeletal traction through Crutchfield tongs (Fig. 2.7) or Gardner-wells tongs | No urgency<br>Only maintenance of reduction of skeletal traction. |
| ↓ | |
| 10 lb weight for head, 5 lb weight for each vertebra to a maximum of 40 lb. | |

If reduction is obtained, weight is ↓by 50 percent. If reduction is not obtained, open reduction is attempted.

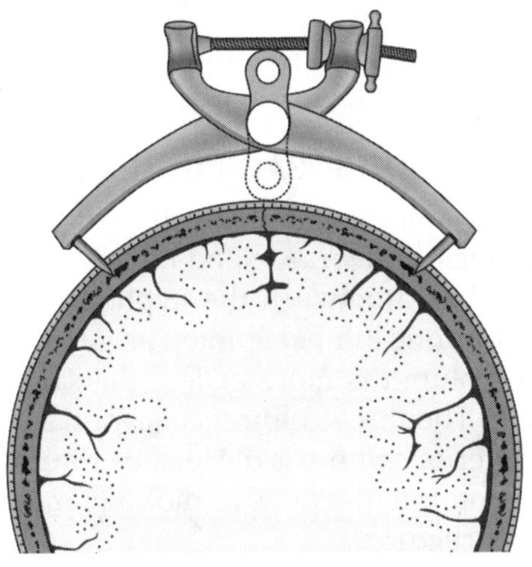

**Fig. 2.7:** Crutchfield tongs

- Anterior decompression consists of removal of the disk and is recommended when disk prolapse is present.
- Anterior cervical plating allows for immediate rigid fixation after decompression and bone grafting. The plates used are H-type or Caspar plates. Recently cervical spine locking plate (CSLP) and reflex anterior cervical plate are providing better fixation and faster rehabilitation.

- Posterior approach preferred for ligamentous instability. Posterior stabilization and rigid internal fixation is provided by systems like Roy-Camillie, Magerl and Seemann, etc. which have posterior plates and screws, hook plates, etc.
- Anterior approach and corpectomy (removal of the crushed body) for burst fracture with cord compression. After corpectomy, a bone graft or a cage fills up the gap.
- Combined anterior and posterior decompression for posterior instability and anterior compression of the neural elements.

Laminectomy has limited role in the treatment of cervical fracture.

Lateral mass screw fixation provides rigid internal fixation in previous laminectomies or when the spinous processes are damaged, etc.

## THORACIC AND LUMBOSACRAL SPINE INJURIES

Thoracolumbar spine is generally regarded as extending from 10th thoracic vertebrae to 2nd lumbar vertebrae and is the transitional area between the kyphotic upper thoracic spines to the lordotic lumbar spine. The general anatomy of the vertebral column is more or less the same as in other areas of spine. The three-column concept has already been described. Anterior column is the load bearing structure and the posterior column functions as motion limiters as well as load bearing structures.

Mercifully, the thoracolumbar injuries spare the upper limbs and vital functions. Though a lesser challenge than cervical injury, nevertheless it poses problems, no less risky than the former.

### Mechanism of Injury

- Fall from a height.
- RTA: Seat belt injury (chance fracture).
- Other causes like gunshot injuries, assault, etc.

**McAfee's Classification—3-column Classification** (Figs 2.8A to D) (For medical readers)

*Wedge Compression*

Isolated failure of anterior column due to forward flexion. No neurological deficit.

*Stable Burst Fractures*

Anterior and middle columns fail. No loss of integrity of posterior elements.

*Unstable Burst Fractures*

Anterior and middle column fail in compression. Posterior column fail in compression, lateral flexion or rotation. Post-traumatic kyphosis and neural symptoms are present.

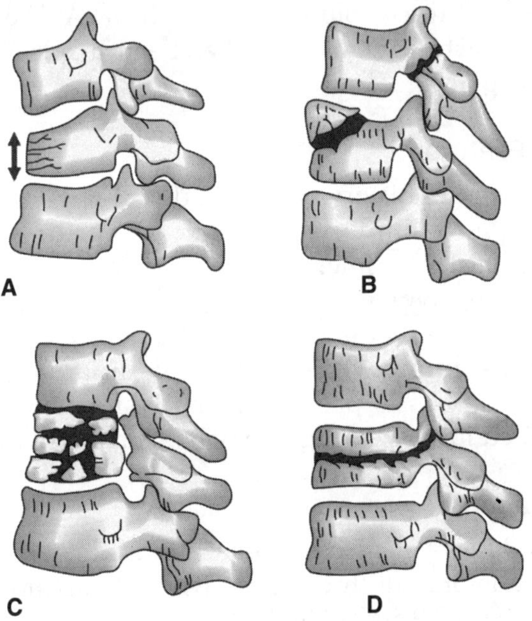


**Figs 5.8A to D:** Thoracolumbar fractures: (A) Wedge compression, (B) Stable burst fracture, (C) Unstable burst fracture, (D) Chance fracture

### *Chance Fracture (Seatbelt Injury)*

It is seen in people who wear a lap belt without a shoulder harness. Horizontal avulsion fracture of vertebral bodies caused by flexion about an axis anterior to the anterior longitudinal ligament. A strong tensile force pulls entire vertebrae apart.

### *Flexion Distraction Injury*

Flexion axis is posterior to the anterior longitudinal ligament. Anterior column fails in compression. Middle and posterior columns fail in tension. It is unstable because supraspinous, interspinous and ligamentum flavum fail.

### *Translational Injuries*

Malalignment of neural canal, which has been totally disrupted. All three columns fail in shear. At the affected level, one part of sacral canal has been displaced in the transverse plane.

## Clinical Features

The patient gives history of trauma due to RTA or fall from a height and complains of pain; posterior swelling, tenderness, palpable interspinous gap or a step may be felt. Neurological involvement may vary from paraplegia to individual nerve root involvement. Spinal shock is present for 24 hours during which all the reflexes are lost. Cauda equina paralysis is present if the lesion is below $L_1$. Exaggerated lumbar lordosis may be seen in old cases.

## Investigations

*Radiography of the affected spine* this is the preliminary investigation and all three views (AP, lateral and oblique) are taken (Figs 2.9 and 2.10). Fracture of the vertebral body, pedicles, lumbar transverse process, pedicles spinous process, etc. is looked for. Disk space and neural canal narrowing is looked for. With the advent of MRI and CT

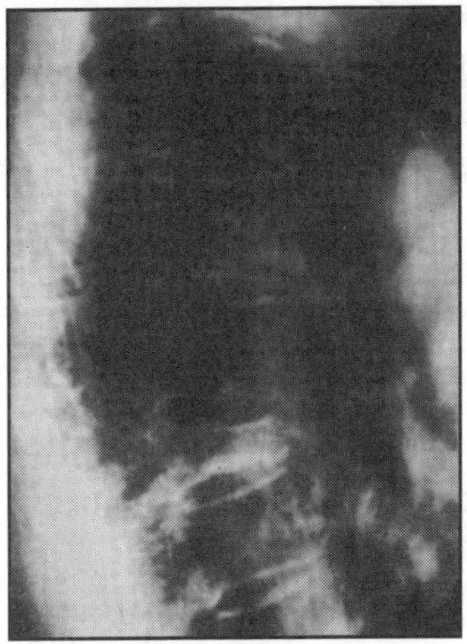

**Fig. 2.9:** Radiograph showing flexion compression fracture of T12 vertebra

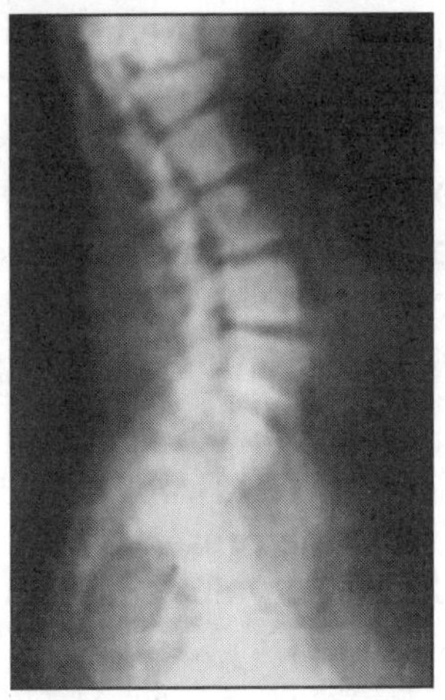

**Fig. 2.10:** Radiograph showing exaggerated lumbar lordosis due to L1 fracture

scan, the role of radiography appears to be diminishing in importance.

*CT scan and MRI* are found to be more useful than radiographs in evaluation of spinal trauma. While CT scan helps in studying the bony elements, MRI helps in the study of both bone and soft tissue elements. The damage to the cord is detected accurately and is now being considered as the "gold standard" in the investigation of spine injury.

**Mystifying Facts: Radiological clues about an unstable spine**

- Loss of vertebral height > 50 percent.
- Kyphosis > 30 percent.
- Spondylolisthesis > 3 mm.

## Management

This is discussed under two heads.

***Management at the site of accident:*** This consists of careful handling of the patient suspected to have spine injury.

Consider all patients with spine injury to have neurological damage, shift them to the hospital with utmost care, and caution avoiding all unnecessary movements.

***Definitive treatment at the hospital:*** The examination and the management measures practiced at the casuality are as follows:

*Practice:* Caution in handling the neck.

*Examination:* The general condition and other systems like CNS/CVS/RS/PA/GI tract, etc. Also, examine from head to toe, the presence of other fractures, head, chest injuries, blunt injury abdomen and pelvic fractures.

*Evaluate:* The spine injury by gentle careful clinical examination. This has to be supplemented by proper investigations like X-ray, CT-scan, MRI, etc.

*Assess:* Carefully assess the level and extent of neurological damage by examining the dermatome, myotome and reflexes.

*Plan:* After evaluating and assessing the damage, plan the line of treatment. The treatment options include nonoperative, traction and operative methods. Now let us carefully took into various treatment modalities.

This varies depending upon the nature of injury and the presence or absence of neurological damage (Flow chart 2.1):

- *For stable fracture without neurological deficit* Less than 30 percent anterior wedge, lateral, central compression fracture of the vertebral body is considered as stable fracture. In these injuries, there is no fracture of the posterior cortex of the vertebral body, and there is no disruption of the neural arch.

  *Treatment:* This is essentially conservative and consists of bed rest, NSAIDs and external spine supports like brace, corsets, etc. If the vertebral body compression is less than 30 percent, only corset is used; and if the compression is more than 30 percent but less than 50 percent, a plaster jacket along with a corset is preferred (Fig. 2.11).

**Flow chart 2.1:** Treatment plan for thoracolumbar injuries

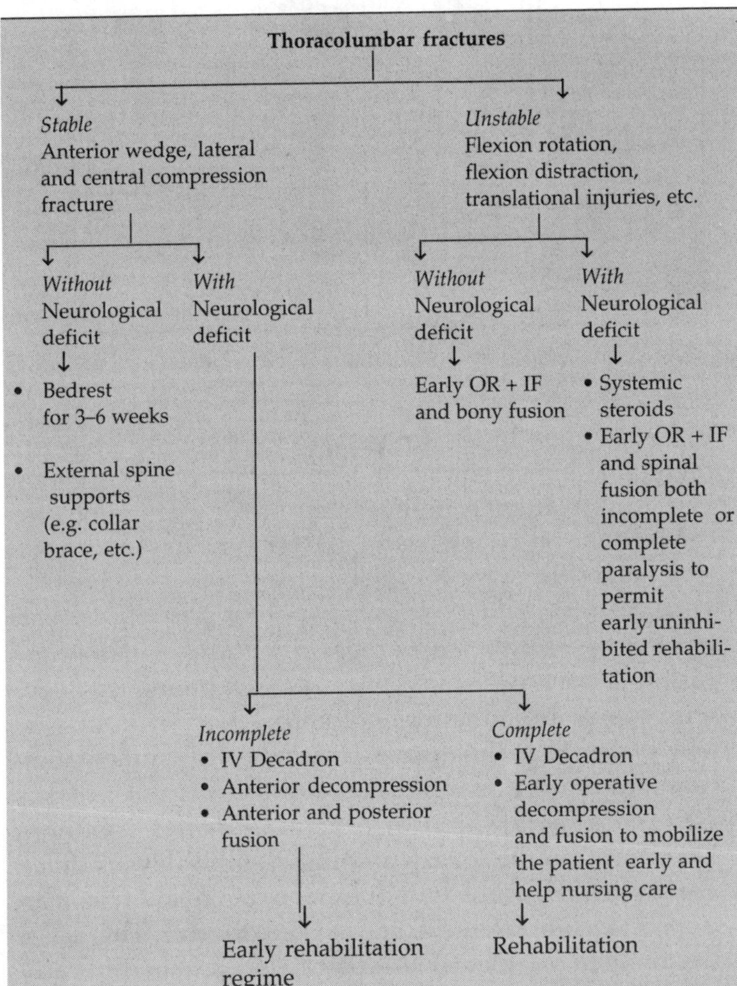


- *For stable fracture with neural deficit:* It has to be first determined whether the neurological deficit is complete (loss of motor power, sensory loss and absent reflexes) or incomplete (only cord or only spinal nerve roots).

  If neurological damage is incomplete, IV steroids are given for 4 days. Anterior decompression and anterior interbody

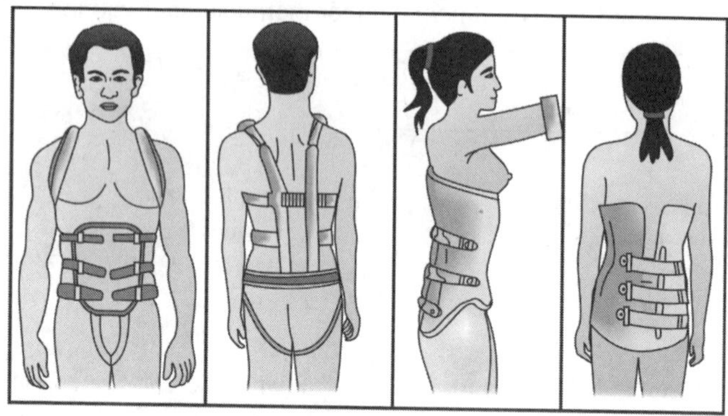

**Fig. 2.11:** Spinal braces for the treatment of stable thoracolumbar injuries

fusion is done in the first stage, followed by posterior segmental spinal stabilization by either pedicle screws, Hart shill rectangle frame, Luque instrumentation, etc. can be done one week later. Laminectomy has fewer roles as it makes the spine less stable.

- *Unstable fracture without neurological deficit:* This is best treated by early open reduction, internal fixation and fusion is done preferably within 12–24 hours. It is done with spinal cord monitoring. Internal fixation is either by VSP plates, Hart shill frame, Harrington instrumentation, titanium cages, etc (Figs 2.12A and B).
- *Unstable fracture with neurological deficit:* Systemic Decadron 4–6 mg/every 6 hours IV for 3 days is given. Early open reduction and internal fixation and fusion are done in incomplete neurological deficit cases. This is also desirable in complete neurological deficit to permit early-uninhibited rehabilitation. Segmental spinal stabilization with Luque or Hart shill frame is recommended.

### Fixation Choices

*Posterior spinal instrumentation* for lumbar fractures: Luque screw segmental spinal instrumentation is found to be very effective.

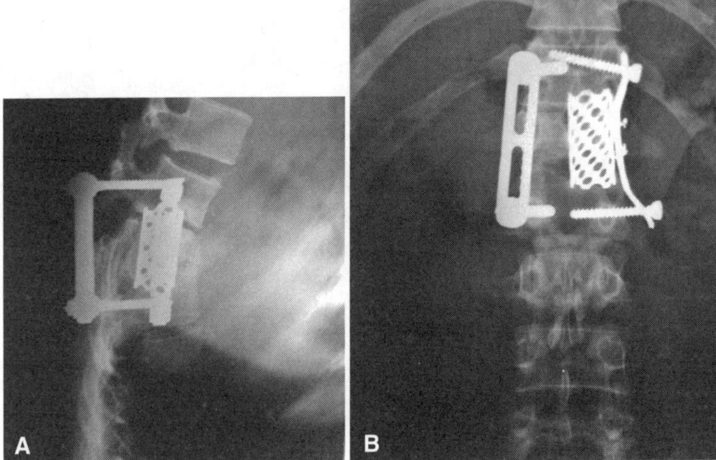

**Figs 2.12A and B:** (A) Radiograph showing posterior instrumentation (Lateral view) Fixation with cage, (B) AP view

*Anterior spinal instrumentation* for fractures from $T_{10}$ to $L_3$ and used as a lateral vertebral body device. However, the procedure is more morbid and is associated with dangerous complications like vascular injury, etc. Anterior plate system can be used to manage the thoracolumbar burst fracture and strut grafts can easily be placed with this approach.

*Anterior vertebral body excison:* This is indicated in vertebral burst fractures of more than two weeks duration and who are not a candidate for posterior instrumentation. This is followed by strut grafting and internal fixation.

# Index

## Clinical Notes

# Clinical Notes

## Clinical Notes

# Clinical Notes